The Food Prescription
for Better Health

**A Cardiologist's Proven Method to Reverse
Heart Disease, Diabetes, Obesity, and
Other Chronic Illnesses, Naturally!**

Baxter D. Montgomery, MD

The Food Prescription
for Better Health

**A Cardiologist's Proven Method to Reverse Heart
Disease, Diabetes, Obesity, and
Other Chronic Illnesses, Naturally!**

By
Baxter D. Montgomery, MD

Delworth Publishing
Houston, Texas
2011

Delworth Publishing
10480 Main Street
Houston, TX 77025
713-599-1144 phone   713-599-1199 fax
delworthpublishing@drbaxtermontgomery.com

ISBN: 0983128715
ISBN-13: 978-0-9831287-1-7
LCCN: 2011921287

Notice
This book is intended as a reference volume only, not as a medical manual. The information given here is designed to help you make informed decisions about your health. It is not intended as a substitute for any treatment that may have been prescribed by your doctor. If you suspect that you have a medical problem, we urge you to seek competent medical help.

Internet addresses and telephone numbers given in this book were accurate at the time it went to press.

༺༻

Editor and Compiler — Kathy Stuesser
Book Packager and Project Coordinator — Rita Mills
Jacket and Graphics Creation — Vicki Mark
Cover Photo — Doug Carter
Text Design — Rita Mills
Illustrations — Baxter D. Montgomery

www.DrBaxterMontgomery.com

Praise for The Food Prescription for Better Health

This is a very important book, both for general practitioners and for patients, and it needs to be in the waiting room of every doctor's office in the country. Dr. Montgomery writes from his heart because he really cares about his patients. Skip the drug store, get this book and you will have the best of all prescriptions!

—T. Colin Campbell, PhD,
Cornell Professor Emeritus and
Best Selling author of The China Study.

Modern cardiology has failed. Coronary bypass and stenting has been demonstrated in meta-analysis to do almost nothing to extend lifespan and protect against future heart attacks. Now we have evidence to demonstrate heart disease can be prevented and even reversed through nutritional interventions, averting future heart attacks. Dr. Montgomery is the cardiologist leading the charge to a new standard of practice—one that saves lives. Imagine if cardiologists all over America taught their patients about nutritional excellence as a means of treating heart disease? It would save an untold amount of suffering and human tragedy.

—Joel Fuhrman, MD
Author of Eat To Live and Eat For Health
Board, American College of Lifestyle Medicine,
Research Director, Nutritional Research Project.

Food Prescription for Better Health *defines a proven lifestyle pathway for enhanced well being and elimination of disease. This must read contribution of Dr. Baxter Montgomery reaffirms that correctly chosen foods are our most powerful medicine.*

—Caldwell B. Esselstyn, Jr., M.D.
Author Prevent and Reverse Heart Disease
Consultant Cleveland Clinic Wellness Institute

Dr. Baxter Montgomery is an experienced, outstanding cardiologist who has taken his vast knowledge in preventing heart disease and put it into his new book, The Food Prescription for Better Health. This book is a "must read" for patients and physicians! It is a well written, easily understood way to achieve optimal health and quality of life. Thanks to Dr. Montgomery for sharing his valuable insights.

—Dan Wolterman
President/CEO Memorial Hermann

Dr. Montgomery is a dedicated and informed cardiologist that walks his talk. A pioneer in disease reversal, he has now put the phenomenal results of his Boot Camp workshops into The Food Prescription for Better Health. This book offers a sensible and natural dietary program designed to restore your health, your awareness, and your hope.

—Verne Varona
Author, Nature's Cancer-Fighting Foods

Dr. Montgomery is ahead of his time. I truly believe that a plant-based, whole food, minimally processed diet will be the norm in 20 years. In today's American culture, it seems radical. I would characterize it as cutting edge. Dr. Montgomery's background in biochemistry as an undergraduate student and in medicine for his profession equip him with a unique perspective to see our food as an agent that can powerfully alter our health. The Food Prescription for Better Health walks you through how to make the transition to a new way of nourishing your body. More that it is a personal story of one man's mission to change the way we think about and consume food.

—Karen Eggert, M.Ed.
Nutrition Enthusiast & Exercise Physiologist

Dr. Montgomery has written a book for individuals from all walks of life. I urge all of my patients and friends to read this book as it presents a very concise "prescription" for good health. Not only does the information in this book benefit patients with cardiovascular disease and diabetes, but those with chronic eye disease. We as physicians must urge our patients not to settle for the simple answer found on a prescription pad, but to strive to find the underlying cause of their illness if they expect a permanent solution.

—Allan J. Panzer, B.S. O.D.
Houston Dry Eye Clinic

෩

Table of Contents

Dedication

I wrote this book in honor of my late mother, Johnsie Lee Montgomery, and father, Aubary Lee Montgomery, who taught me many things in life through their actions as loving parents. Although I have had the pleasure to work with many bright individuals in my lifetime, including Nobel Laureates, Rhode scholars, and numerous MDs and PhDs, I have met no one as wise and insightful as my mother and father.

I also dedicate this book to my older brother and sister, Don and Judy, for their love and support for me throughout my life. They have "been there" for me through "thick and thin," and remain dedicated siblings.

Lastly, I dedicate this book to my four beautiful children—Baxter Jr., Suzette A., Aleigha, and Zoewye. Because of them, the sun is brighter, the sky is bluer, and the air is fresher. I thank God for placing them in my life.

◦〜

Acknowledgments

No significant work is the sole creation of a single individual, and this book is no exception. First, and foremost, I thank the Lord for His divine intervention. I do not think I could have even begun this effort in the setting of all the challenges in my life at the time of this writing without Him.

Special thanks go to the many clients and patients who participated in the different Nutritional Boot Camps and gave their valuable feedback. I appreciate the work of Brittanee Jones and Sean Johnson, for their efforts in tracking the data of wellness clients and clinical patients who participated in the Nutritional Boot Camps. I also want to grant special acknowledgment to Odalys Valdivia for over eleven years of hard work and dedication to the medical office, as her efforts have been institutional.

I thank the following individuals for their past and ongoing dedicated service to Montgomery Heart and Wellness: Edie Andress, Ingrid Brade, Vanessa Washington, Amanda Petrie, Darlonda Bradshaw, Tameka Roberson, and Barbara Brown. A special thanks to Rashme Patel and Kala Asante for their valuable volunteer work.

I appreciate the work of Beverly Shirkey, for her timely and detailed statistical analysis of our data. Karen Eggert contributed greatly to the content of the Nutritional Boot Camp and the critique of the Food Classification System. Anasa Blackman and Cheryl Pradia contributed to the food preparation demonstrations and recipe development.

Special thanks go to Ayesha Kabir and John Sampson for their efforts in researching the documentation, critiquing the food classification system, and developing recipes and menus.

Also, thanks to Ari Pramudji and Matthew Robinson for helping to refine the food classification system. Finally, thank you Kathy Stuesser for your creativity, insight, and overall moral support. You provided valuable editing, critiquing, and organizing efforts towards this book. Working with you has been a true blessing.

❧

Foreword

When you visit a doctor's office, you expect to leave with a prescription. If you have an infection, you'll get an antibiotic. If you have high cholesterol, you'll be sent off to the pharmacy for a bottle of statin drugs. Dr. Baxter Montgomery has a prescription, too. But it is in many ways more powerful than drugs could ever be.

In North America and much of the rest of the world, less-than-healthful eating habits have led to out-of-control rates of health problems. Conditions that were once seen only in adults are now cropping up at alarming rates in children. One in five American teenagers already has an abnormal cholesterol level. A third of children are either overweight or obese. And one in three children born since the year 2000 will develop diabetes at some point in life.

A change in eating habits can change all this. Our research at the Physicians Committee for Responsible Medicine has shown that a plant-based diet can help you lose weight and dramatically improve your health. It is gratifying to see the extent to which people are able to tackle type 2 diabetes, cholesterol problems, high blood pressure, and long-standing weight challenges.

Even though a plant-based diet elicits more pronounced nutritional changes than less far-reaching diets, they turn out to be surprisingly easy to follow. And a healthy diet is so rewarding, you'll never want to let it go. Leading health organizations now support plant-based diets for all stages of life. The American Dietetic Association, American Diabetes Association, and others point out the benefits these diets have and the body of scientific evidence that supports their use.

Dr. Montgomery has devoted his career to developing a comprehensive prescription for good nutrition that could save your life. In the following pages, Dr. Montgomery shares the healthiest types of foods to choose and the healthiest food preparation methods. And he makes it practical, classifying foods based on their ability to heal—or harm—our bodies, taking into account food processing, chemical characteristics, and other properties. It all starts with a Nutrition Boot Camp. But don't worry— most people find it to be a breeze, and will be thrilled as they feel its wide-ranging health benefits.

In his clinical practice and through his educational efforts, Dr. Montgomery is spreading the word that the foods we consume can dramatically affect our health and how we function from day to day. He is inspiring us to make real changes in our lives. And he goes further, encouraging us to set healthful traditions for future generations. After reading this book, I would suggest that you share it with your loved ones and anyone interested in taking control of their health. If everyone followed this book's visionary advice, it could revolutionize the health of the planet.

Neal Barnard, M.D., is a nutrition researcher and president of the Physicians Committee for Responsible Medicine. He is also the author of *Breaking the Food Seduction* and *Dr. Neal Barnard's Program for Reversing Diabetes*.

ᖇ

Preface

America's health care system is one of the hottest topics debated today. We as a society are concerned about skyrocketing costs, reductions in services, and burdens placed on the system to cover emergency needs of the uninsured. We spend incredible amounts of money annually to get the best health care we can afford. With all the money we throw at it, we should expect to be some of the healthiest people in the world. Sadly, that is not the case. We keep spending more money, only to find ourselves getting sicker. It feels at times like we are paying to become ill! I have now spent many years practicing internal medicine, cardiology, and cardiac electrophysiology. During this time, I have witnessed amazing advances in medical science. Despite these advances, I have seen more young people than ever before, plagued by chronic illnesses.

As a medical student in the late 1980s, my patients with conditions such as type 2 diabetes, hypertension, obesity, high cholesterol, or arthritis, were typically in their sixth or seventh decade of life. Now, I frequently see adolescents, teens, and young adults with these same conditions. I noticed over time that I was becoming sicker as well. My LDL cholesterol had risen to 138 by the age of 38. It should have been less than 100 mg/dL. As a cardiologist with a genetic predisposition to diabetes and heart disease, I knew this was a significant problem.

I began an intense research effort, looking for alternative ways to achieve optimal health and wellness. In my search, I discovered a simple but amazing fact—when it comes to disease reversal and prevention, nutritional excellence is everything.

Unfortunately, too few doctors consider nutrition as a means to restore good health. Drug companies work hard to convince us all that curing illness starts in the pharmacy section of the grocery store, not the produce department. When someone becomes ill, health care professionals are trained to offer a drug or surgery to get them well. Collectively, we think of medications as near cure-alls. This is simply not the truth!

Often, what is really going on with such treatments is just the masking of symptoms. Chronic illnesses, and acute illnesses for that matter, are primarily due to biochemical and physiological imbalances. Studies have shown that chronic illnesses are the direct result of our poor lifestyle choices, the most damaging of which is our food choices. We eat too many unnatural, processed foods that are toxic to our bodies, in place of foods that are natural and supply what our bodies need.

We need a paradigm shift in our approach to healthcare. Our efforts need to start with removing unnatural foods from our diet, and replacing those foods with ones that are "natural," as a way of reversing illness and facilitating health. This new approach would be a shift away from the standard approach of using medical and surgical interventions as our primary protocols. This fundamental change provides the foundation of *The Food Prescription* I have written for my patients and wellness clients over the years, and now for the general public.

My experience has been that not all patients "take their medicine" willingly. When asked to follow a healthier lifestyle, some immediately become concerned about foods they will be forced to give up. "Doc, what do I have to give up eating?" I ask them in response, "What are you *willing* to give up? What is a good pair of kidneys going for these days? Are you willing to give up your heart or brain? How about your legs?" The foods we eat daily result in the loss of heart, kidney, brain, and liver function. In essence, we are trading our very lives in exchange for the addictive, toxic foods we eat daily. As we strive to become healthier, there needs to be a paradigm shift in the medical community. We need to recognize that many people are able to achieve good health and heal themselves of disease without surgery or drugs. This shows that, with a better understanding of human physiology and nutrition, we can create a healthy, disease-free society just by changing the way we eat.

Why I am Writing This Book

Like many people, I have witnessed close loved ones suffer from chronic illnesses at the end of their lives. The experience of watching what they went through, as well as seeing the compromised qualities of life my patients have endured over the years, has allowed me to "place a face" on the devastation brought about by chronic illnesses. I have as a result of my own careful research and study, developed, and then systemically incorporated food prescriptions into my cardiology practice. The results I have seen first-hand from the experiences of hundreds of patients and clients, across a broad spectrum of health conditions, have been astounding.

I believe this success is the result of two very important factors. First, the biochemical truth of the body's impressive ability to heal itself when provided nutritionally excellent fuel is undeniable. Second, I take a very direct approach in telling individuals how they need to choose and prepare food to improve their health so there is no confusion. We guide individuals through the process, every step of the way.

My mission is now to extend the success that I have seen in my practice to people everywhere. I want people to understand that living a healthier lifestyle is easier than they think, and the rewards are greater than they can even imagine. Run a marathon at 70? Yes. Chase after grandchildren without shortness of breath? Yes. Beat your genetic predisposition to diabetes, heart disease, and cancer? Yes. Your destiny is in your control. My question to you now is, "What are you willing to gain?"

⁓

Chapter One
The Lethal Fork

A 69-year-old woman came into my office during my early years as a cardiologist. She complained of dizziness and memory loss, as well as chronic chest discomfort. She also suffered from diabetes, high blood pressure, was chronically overweight, had elevated cholesterol levels, and carpal tunnel syndrome. She routinely took several medications for these conditions. Although she had significant risk factors for heart disease, I was concerned that the dizziness and memory loss she experienced likely pointed to a neurological (brain) problem, rather than something going on with her heart. A brain MRI revealed a benign tumor that explained both the dizziness and memory loss. She would have to have the tumor removed.

To prepare her for surgery we had to evaluate her heart to determine the extent that her multiple heart disease risk factors and chest pain symptoms might create problems for her during surgery. She had a heart catheterization and coronary angiogram, which revealed a critically narrowed region in an area that supplies blood to about 75% of the left main chamber of her heart. A narrowing in this location is often referred to as the "widow maker," or in this case, potentially a "widower maker." Fortunately, we caught the problem in time and a successful angioplasty and stent placement allowed her to have the tumor near her brain removed after a few months.

Her overall recovery from the procedure was good, and she was discharged home within one to two weeks in good functional condition. A good outcome, right? Unfortunately, this was not the end of the story. Events would later unfold for this patient that would change the focus of my career, forever.

America's Current State of Health

The fact that the patient I just described had multiple concurrent conditions was not unusual. This fact caused me to realize how much sicker my patients were becoming over time. It had become normal to see patients with several major health issues going on at the same time. The news media confirmed this trend went well beyond my practice to the nation at large. I found the gravity of this situation to be profoundly alarming. Obesity, heart disease, cancer, and diabetes had become conditions that we would all be impacted by in some way. As a physician and nutritional advocate, I feel compelled to help people understand the implications of this new reality. So, what is the current state of our health and how is it affecting us?

According to the World Health Organization (WHO), the major risk factors influencing mortality today are our patterns of living and consumption. In countries like the United States, Canada, and Western Europe, people die from complications related to the fact that we simply eat too much, drink too much, and exercise too little.[1] Despite our over consumption of food, our poor health is primarily because of *what* we eat more than *how much* we eat. Our forks have become lethal.

Our eating habits have led to increasing numbers of overweight and clinically obese Americans. This is tragic. We need to view being overweight as a critical sign of deteriorating health. More than mere inconvenience, being overweight is associated with adverse metabolic effects on blood pressure, cholesterol, triglycerides, and insulin resistance. Risks increase greatly for coronary heart disease, ischemic stroke, and type 2 diabetes. Sadly, we often focus primarily on the superficial aspects of being overweight, and miss the core issue that carrying excess weight is really an outward manifestation of inner disease. Being overweight or obese has reached epidemic proportions globally. WHO estimated in 2005 that 1.6 billion adults, age 15 or older, were overweight, and at least 400 million were obese. The organization projects that by the year 2015, 2.5 billion adults globally will be overweight, and another 700 million will be obese.[2] In February 2010, WHO reported that at least 2.6 million people die each year as a result of being overweight or obese.[3] In 2005, WHO estimated there were at least 20 million overweight children under the age of 5, globally. This has to date not been an issue, but now demands the creation of global weight standards that can be used to diagnose unhealthy conditions more quickly.

In April 2006, WHO released new child growth standards that included BMI (body mass index) charts for infants and children under the age of five. For young girls, this raises even more concern. Many studies show that obesity in young girls can lead to early onset of puberty.[4] Other studies show that starting menstrual cycles early increases the risk of breast cancer later in life.[5] Body fat can produce sex hormones, causing girls as young as 7 or 8 years old to develop breasts, which is one of the first signs of puberty. These girls may also start menstrual cycles at an earlier age, which results in their exposure to estrogen and progesterone hormones over a longer span of years. This exposure is what puts them at risk for breast cancer later. This sobering evidence should serve as a wakeup call to the potential broad impacts of our eating habits. We have to realize that poor eating habits do not just affect our health. We are in fact poisoning our children with the standard American diet, turning a blind eye to the problem of childhood obesity, and as a result, subjecting the ones we love to a ripple effect of health and social consequences. We also need to be concerned that we have become a nation of "sitters." Unlike our predecessors, fewer of us perform jobs that require manual labor. We sit in an office behind a desk. We drive more than we walk, even to the extreme of circling parking lots to secure front row parking. We shop on the Internet to avoid walking in malls and have goods delivered to our front door. Our free time is spent in front of the television or computer, rather than playing outdoor sports with our family and friends. We need to find a way to get ourselves up and moving!

The WHO estimates that physical inactivity is responsible for 1.9 million annual deaths, globally, and accounts for 10-16% of the world's cases of breast cancer, colon and rectal cancers, and diabetes. Our failure to get adequate exercise accounts for 22% of cases of ischemic heart disease.

It's possible that our poor diets are contributing to our sedentary lifestyle. One study based on research of animal behavior suggests a diet low in animal protein results in more voluntary exercise.[6] In addition, an unhealthy diet that causes obesity, high blood pressure, and heart disease would not support regular exercise. Hence, our poor exercise habits may actually be the result of our poor diets.

The leading causes of death in this country might not come as a surprise, but the fact that these causes are the result of choices largely within our control may be new information for some. The chart below (Figureure1.1) shows the leading causes of death in the United States in the year 2007.[7] While this data was collected in 2007, it very likely holds true today. Heart disease, or diseases of the heart, is the number one cause of death in the United States, followed by cancer and stroke. Stroke can actually be added to heart disease, because most causes of stroke are due to heart disease-related illnesses. If we combine the remaining disorders on the list beyond heart disease, cancer, and stroke, the sum of these disorders would still not equal the deaths caused by heart disease! Heart disease and cancer are the most common causes of death in America today. What may come as a surprise to many people is that heart disease, cancer, and stroke are considered lifestyle disorders, and are primarily impacted by poor nutrition. The evidence is clear—our standard American diet is killing us!

Figure 1.1

Leading Causes of Death in the U.S. in 2007

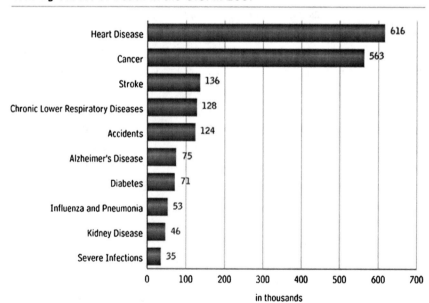

Here are some of the top causes of death in more detail.

Heart and Blood Vessel (Cardiovascular) Disease

> *A man was told that he had a heart attack.*
> *Imagine what you would have to do to your*
> *heart for it to come out of your body and attack*
> *you.*
>
> **—Dick Gregory**

Cardiovascular (*cardio* meaning heart and *vascular* meaning blood vessels) disease has an impact on a wide range of body systems that can result in a number of medical problems and symptoms. Most individuals with this disease see their doctor with problems directly related to the heart. A primary concern is usually chest discomfort (angina), which may be caused by a significant reduction of blood flow to the heart (ischemia), or obstruction of blood flow to parts of the heart (heart attack). Other symptoms may include shortness of breath and swelling, caused by poor overall circulation, and congestion due to a weakened heart.

What are the facts about the hearts of Americans?

Cardiovascular disease statistics from the American Heart Association, based on 2007 data, show some interesting facts:[8]

- Coronary heart disease (CHD) is the leading cause of death in the U.S.
- About 452 million people die each year from CHD.
- 1.26 million Americans are estimated to suffer an initial or recurrent heart attack each year.
- Over 10 million people suffer from angina pectoris—symptoms caused by poor blood circulation to the heart.
- It is estimated that 500,000 new cases of stable angina occur each year.
- 17.6 million people alive today have a history of heart attack, angina pectoris, or both.
- Approximately 7.9 million Americans, age 20 and older have experienced a prior heart attack.

These numbers underscore the fact that Americans are "broken hearted." While statistics are helpful, it is helpful to put a face on the data.[9] On February 11, 2010, former President Bill Clinton presented to his cardiologist with symptoms of chest "discomfort." Now 63 years old, he had undergone a four-vessel coronary artery bypass surgery, six years prior. His cardiologist was so concerned about his symptoms that he recommended Clinton be admitted to the hospital to undergo some tests. A procedure known as a coronary angiogram was done, revealing a blockage of a vein, which was used to bypass one of the originally blocked arteries (the native artery) of the heart. Two stents were placed in the native (original) artery to improve blood flow. Clinton tolerated the angiogram procedure and was released from the hospital the following day.

Former President Bill Clinton's Fight over the years with heart disease is well documented by the media. Various cardiology experts around the country have stated his clinical scenario as typical, and that his condition will only progress over time. They state he will likely develop more "blockages," and will need more procedures. The former President's story underscores the fact that heart disease has no boundaries when it comes to political power, social status, fame, or wealth. Tim Russert, former anchor of *Meet The Press*, and Jim Fixx, a former runner, and author of the 1977 best-seller, *The Complete Book of Running*, both died suddenly from heart attacks in their 50s. When interviewed about the death of Tim Russert, Dr. Cam Patterson, chief of cardiology at the University of North Carolina at Chapel Hill stated, "It's still the leading cause of death and disability. Half the people who are walking around are going to die at some point of heart disease."[10]

> **To An Athlete Dying Young**
> The time you won your town the race
> We chaired you through the market place;
> Man and boy stood cheering by,
> And home we brought you shoulder-high.
> Today, the road all runners come,
> Shoulder-high we bring you home,
> And set you at your threshold down,
> Townsman of a stiller town.
>
> **—A.E. Hausman, 1895**

Fifty years old seems too young to die so suddenly. How young is too young for heart disease?

We mistakenly believe that heart disease is something the old alone bear. However, the review of three pathological studies gives insight into just how common heart disease is in the young.

- A study of 300 American soldiers killed in the Korean War was done to investigate the pathology of coronary artery disease. The subjects of the study were men with an average age of 22.1 years. In 77.3% of the cases, gross evidence of coronary disease was demonstrated.[11]

- A multicenter autopsy study examined the relation of risk factors for adult coronary artery disease to atherosclerosis (plaque inside the walls of the arteries) in nearly 3,000 persons. Subjects ranged in age from 15-34 years, all died from accidents, homicides, or suicides, and all were autopsied in forensic laboratories. The study showed that raised levels of fatty plaques were seen in individuals as young as 15 years old. These raised plaques were associated with elevated cholesterol, diabetes, increased BMI, and smoking. [12]

- A study conducted by researchers at the Department of Medicine, University of Louisville, Kentucky, involved 111 victims of non-cardiac trauma. Their study population involved primarily white males (86.4%), with a mean age of 26 +/- 6 years. Their report showed coronary artery disease was present in 78% in this group.[13] These studies clearly reveal that heart disease starts very young for Americans, and is seen in high numbers for people we would not ordinarily expect. Given the current high levels of obesity and type 2 diabetes in American adolescents and young adults, we would easily expect to get the same high levels of coronary artery disease today in young people as was found in the study of American soldiers killed in the Korean War. This evidence alone leads us to suspect that as Americans reach their fifth and sixth decades of life, heart disease may in fact be a universal condition.

Cancer

> *Dear God, I pray for the cure of cancer. Amen.*
> *Going along for years in remission, and then one day it pops its head up again. If you ever have it, you will never be free of it. Pray for the day there will be a permanent cure.*
>
> **—Anonymous**

This prayer was sent to me in an email. It could have originated from a cancer survivor who suffered a recurrence of cancer, or perhaps was from a family member or other loved one. Regardless of its origin, it echoes the sentiment that many individuals in our society feel. Personal experience, family members, friends, neighbors, or simply admired public figures—nearly all of us have been touched by cancer in one way or another. Cancer has an unusual "sticking factor," in that individuals who suffer from this disease often suffer for long periods while living with the disease. Prolonged chemotherapy treatments, hair and weight loss, vomiting, and pain syndromes frequently become "life partners" of the cancer victim. We commonly talk about cancer as a single disease. While this is biologically true, cancer clinically behaves as a family of diseases that vary based on the organ or tissue it affects. Its clinical course can range from a slow growing, chronically benign condition, to a rapidly progressive lethal one. Therefore, any meaningful discussion on cancer must focus on the organ or tissue it affects. Our discussion on cancer will focus on the most prevalent cancer types diagnosed in the United States—lung, colorectal, breast, and prostate.

Lung Cancer

I was working a rotation in an emergency department of a local hospital as a fourth-year medical student when a middle-aged female came in, complaining of a persistent cough and a twenty-pound weight loss over a period of two months. She denied having any fever or chills. She was a chronic smoker. Her blood tests showed an elevated white blood count, which is a sign that her body's immune system had been activated to fight something. She was at the same time anemic. The diagnosis was obvious—lung cancer.

> *Now that I'm gone, I tell you— Don't smoke, whatever you do, just don't smoke. If I could take back that smoking, we wouldn't be talking about any cancer. I'm convinced of that.*
>
> **—Yul Brenner**

What are the facts about Lung Cancer?

According to the National Lung Cancer Partnership:[14]

- Approximately 219,000 people are diagnosed with lung cancer in the U.S. each year—over 103,000 women and nearly 116,000 men.
- Lung cancer kills more than 160,000 people annually—more people than breast, colon, and prostate cancers *combined.*
- Lung cancer is responsible for more than 28% of all cancer related deaths each year.
- Smoking is the primary cause of lung cancer. Approximately 87% of lung cancer cases occur in people who are currently smoking or have previously smoked.
- Although the risk of developing lung cancer goes down with smoking cessation, a significant risk remains for 20 years or longer after quitting.
- Roughly, 84% of people diagnosed with lung cancer die within five years of their diagnosis, compared to 11% of breast cancer, and less than 1% of prostate cancer patients.

Dana Reeve was famous as the wife of Christopher Reeve, best known for his role of Superman and for his tragic spinal cord injury that eventually claimed his life. Dana Reeve took over as chairperson of the Christopher Reeve foundation after his death, and remained committed to spinal cord research until her death at 44 from lung cancer.[15] Dana Reeve never smoked. Her story should serve as a reminder that a chronic disease state is not always (if ever) simply linked to a single adverse lifestyle action. It is likely related to a complex set of conditions that result in the body not functioning optimally and resulting in the development of disease.

Colorectal Cancer

By definition, colorectal cancer is cancer of the large intestine (colon), including its last seven inches (the rectum). Most cases of colon cancer begin as small, noncancerous (benign) clumps of cells, called adenomatous polyps. Over time, some of these polyps become colon cancers. Polyps may be small and produce few, if any, symptoms. For this reason, regular screening tests are recommended to help "prevent" colon cancer by identifying polyps before they become cancerous. The problem I have with the above statement is that it considers polyps to be "noncancerous" or "precancerous." These polyps represent the manifestation of a "cancerous condition" that has been present for years or even decades. Our screening colonoscopies can only detect late stages of the "colorectal cancer condition." To protect ourselves fully from the dangers of colon cancer, we need to view the presence of any polyps as a warning that something is wrong with our body's natural biochemistry or physiology. This outcome should immediately prompt us to focus on better nutrition, specifically eating only natural plant-based foods.

What are the facts about Colorectal Cancer?

In the year 2006:[16]
- 139,127 people were diagnosed with colorectal cancer.
- 53,196 people in the United States died of colorectal cancer.
- Colorectal cancer is the second leading cause of cancer-related deaths in the United States.
- Only 61% of adults aged 50 years or older reported having received a screening occult blood test.

Breast Cancer

Susan G. Komen became the face of breast cancer after she lost her own battle to the disease. Before she died, Susan asked her sister Nancy Brinker to do something to help other women avoid suffering her same fate.[17] The Susan G. Komen Breast Cancer Foundation was born out of that request in 1982 and has since generated over $750 million for breast cancer research. The foundation has touched nearly every scientific advance in breast cancer over the past 20 years.

What are the facts about Breast Cancer?

Not counting some kinds of skin cancer, breast cancer in the United States has the following characteristics:[18]

- It is the most common cancer in women, no matter your race or ethnicity.
- It is the most common cause of death from cancer among Hispanic women.
- It is the second most common cause of death from cancer among white, black, Asian/Pacific Islander, and American Indian/Alaska Native women.

In 2006:
- 191,410 women were diagnosed with breast cancer.
- 40,820 women died from breast cancer.

Nancy Brinker did much, starting as a single voice to change how breast cancer is diagnosed and treated in this country. This shows the power of one lone voice that can rise above the noise in our busy lives and start a movement that ultimately benefits millions of people. I have that same kind of passion for the power of nutrition to change people's lives, and my hope is that I, too, can start a movement that convinces people to employ healthy eating as a new way of life.

Prostate Cancer

The prostate is a gland that helps store seminal fluid. Prostate cancer often begins with symptoms of urinary discomfort or urinary abnormalities, such as the frequency of urination or difficulty in passing urine.

There is a high prevalence of prostate cancer seen on autopsy studies of elderly men, age greater than 75 years old, who die of other causes.[19] The question that is frequently raised is whether prostate cancer is a disease or a natural progression of aging. It is my strong opinion that prostate cancer, like heart disease, diabetes, and other chronic illnesses is a disease that becomes more common with prolonged exposure to poor nutrition. Prostate cancer, generally speaking, is a slow growing cancer in which men will often live with the disease for years, and perhaps decades before dying of some condition, usually other than prostate cancer. Like with other chronic illnesses, the concern with prostate cancer has more to do with living with the disease, as opposed to dying from it.

What are the Facts about Prostate Cancer?

Not counting some forms of skin cancer, prostate cancer in the United States is:[20]

- The most common cancer in men, no matter your race or ethnicity.
- The second most common cause of death from cancer among white, African American,
- American Indian/Alaska Native, and Hispanic men.
- The fourth most common cause of death from cancer among Asian/Pacific Islander men.
- More common in African-American men compared to white men.
- Less common in American Indian/Alaska Native and Asian/Pacific Islander men compared to white men.
- More common in Hispanic men compared to non-Hispanic men.

In 2006:

- 203,415 men developed prostate cancer. (Statistic covers 96% of U.S. population.)
- 28,372 men died from prostate cancer. (Statistic covers 100% of U.S. population.)

The Rest of the Story

The patient I introduced earlier, a person who had such a profound impact on my career, would have benefited by receiving a Food Prescription earlier in her treatment. After returning home, my patient developed hydrocephalus. This is a condition where fluid collects within the brain, secondary to the meningitis that occurred after surgery. This required a brain shunt to be placed to treat this condition. The brain shunt procedure resulted in bleeding in the brain, leading to a one-week coma. She recovered from the coma with frequent seizures and a residual aphasia—a condition consisting of an impaired ability to express or understand language. After extensive rehabilitation and hospitalization, she made a significant recovery, only to decline further after a fall resulted in a second brain bleed. She required an emergent procedure to drain blood from around the brain, and more prolonged hospitalization on life support. At this point, she developed abdominal swelling, secondary to liver failure. Despite more surgery and hospitalization, she died as a result of liver failure, approximately one year and ten months after her initial surgery. Why did she suffer a prolonged illness and eventual death despite such advanced medical and surgical therapy? She had the best that "healthcare" could offer but suffered miserably before dying. After careful review of this patient's medical condition, it became clear that her clinical demise began long before her diagnosis of a meningioma. Evidence of her liver dysfunction could be found, long before her last weeks of life, and was likely brought about by a chronic exposure to processed foods and medications known to contribute to liver dysfunction.

There were many significant characteristics of this patient's condition. The most significant to me was that she was my mother. As I observed her condition during her final days, I recognized clinical factors that were helpful for many of my other patients. One major thing is that her chronic illness preceded her clinical diagnosis of meningioma. Her health condition was on a steady decline, long before her initial hospitalization. For years, she was part of a group I refer to as "the walking ill." Individuals whose underlying illnesses go undiagnosed because they do not have outward signs or symptoms of disease typify the walking ill. *Food Prescription* will describe how optimal nutrition can prevent, arrest, or reverse many chronic illnesses, at any stage. These basic insights have helped me treat and reverse serious conditions of many patients since my mother's death. Furthermore, her death was the impetus for my intense research into natural approaches to disease reversal. My knowledge in this field continues to grow.

My mother impacted me in many ways throughout my life. Perhaps most important was through her teaching. She taught me how to "tell time" on a clock, how to read and spell. She helped me learn my spelling words in fifth grade, and Latin vocabulary in high school and college. She encouraged my youthful inquisitive nature to learn more and to become better. She would often tell me, "Son, I'm going to be your mother until the day I die." I never knew how prophetic this statement would be. It was on her dying bed that she, as a dutiful mother, essentially taught me the most important lesson in clinical medicine of my career.

The experience of watching what my mother went through, as well as seeing the compromised qualities of life my patients endure has forever changed me. My desire to convey the importance of nutrition and its role to allow my patients and the general public to live better lives has evolved from a passion to a personal ministry. The widespread suffering from conditions as relatively minor as headaches, sinus congestion, and impotence, to more major conditions, such as heart disease, cancer, stroke, and lung disease need not be. The current healthcare crisis that has a paralyzing grip on the US economy can be released. We, in fact have control over the very factors that place us at risk! Our standard American diet is what puts our health at risk for these and other diseases. The sooner we take action to change our poor eating choices, the sooner our bodies can heal and reverse these disease states. This is something to celebrate!

ᔕ

The True Origin of Chronic Illness

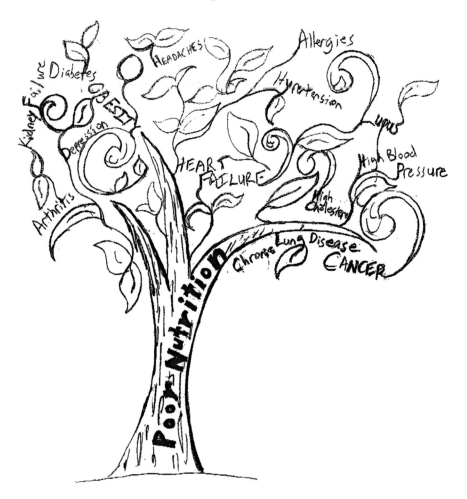

Poor nutrition supports chronic illnesses as the tree trunk supports the tree. The definitive treatment for any chronic illness requires removing its base of poor nutrition, allowing for future growth of health and well being.

Chapter Two
Today's Menu—Tomorrow's Chronic Disease

In the last chapter, we learned that heart disease and cancer are two of the top three causes of death in America. These diseases can be fatal, but we cannot ignore the long-term damaging effects of these and other chronic conditions, existing for years or decades, and limiting our quality of life and stealing our joy. The Centers for Disease Control defines chronic diseases as non-communicable diseases that are prolonged in duration, and do not resolve spontaneously, or are not cured completely.[1] The top chronic diseases in the United States are heart disease and stroke, cancer, diabetes, arthritis, and obesity.

In the United States, chronic diseases cause seven in ten deaths each year. Approximately one in two American adults live with at least one chronic illness. More than 75% of our health care costs in this country are due to chronic conditions, and one-fourth of persons living with chronic illnesses experience significant limitations in daily activities. Rates of chronic illness for children have also been on the rise with approximately 7% of children and adolescents diagnosed with chronic illnesses in 2004, which is up from 1.8 %, estimated back in the 1960s.

The irony of chronic diseases is that they are the most common and most costly of all health problems in America, while at the same time being the most preventable. The CDC identifies four common habits that are damaging but modifiable behaviors that influence chronic diseases. These behaviors are:
- Tobacco use
- Excessive alcohol use
- Insufficient physical activity
- Poor eating habits

We need to face the reality that while 50% of American adults suffer from at least one chronic illness, we also hold in our hands the key to avoiding this outcome! We need to take ownership for making better choices to help ourselves and the people we love. We have come to accept the first two causes of chronic disease—tobacco use and excessive drinking—to be the most damaging lifestyle choices. Certainly, these habits are tied to life-threatening diseases, like lung cancer, emphysema, cirrhosis of the liver, and more. Nevertheless, data from the CDC showing the extent of these habits fall short of fully explaining the widespread nature of chronic illnesses in this country.

According to the CDC, one in six adolescents and adults is a binge drinker. One in five American adults and high school students use tobacco products. Even combined, these destructive habits do not account for why 50% of Americans suffer from chronic illnesses.

Now let's look at the remaining two common habits leading to chronic illness—insufficient physical activity and poor eating habits. The CDC estimates that 60% of adults, as well as adolescents and children live a sedentary lifestyle. Almost two-thirds of Americans get little or no physical exercise on a regular basis!

Apparently, the exercise we are getting involves covering the distance between the sofa and refrigerator, over and over, and over again. Poor dietary habits, such as eating large amounts of saturated fat, are seen in more than 60% of U.S. children and adolescents. An astounding 76% of adults and 80% of high school students in this country do not receive adequate servings of fruits and vegetables. We may feel that we are making better choices when we do not smoke or drink alcohol excessively, and we are. However, we must realize that the poor eating habits and maintaining sedentary lifestyles are the primary reasons we suffer from chronic illnesses.

We have all been told our entire lives that eating well and exercising are keys to health. What may be new for some is the idea that these same good habits do more than promote health—they protect us from chronic illness.

However, between the habits of eating well and exercising, which does more to protect us against chronic illness? In general, people who suffer from high cholesterol, diabetes, obesity, and hypertension often maintain these chronic disorders despite getting regular exercise. It is only when they nourish their bodies properly that they get significant results. Therefore, poor nutrition trumps tobacco, alcohol, and sedentary lifestyles as the primary cause for the development of chronic illnesses. We cannot ignore the reality that what we eat is totally within our control, and our choices are what determine the level of risk we have of becoming ill. To understand what is at stake, we will take a closer look at some of the more common chronic disorders.

Obesity

A woman who had followed our nutritional regimen for a number of months came into my office one day, distressed that her mother and aunt had become concerned about the amount of weight she had lost. They felt she had lost too much weight and looked sickly. Her family was worried for her health, despite the fact that her body mass index was well within the normal range.

It occurred to me after she left that being overweight or even obese in this country had reached a point where people considered these conditions normal. Although this young woman had improved her overall health condition by reversing her obesity, her family members felt she was worse off. They were so accustomed to seeing her overweight that they found her new, normal physique strange, and were ready to label her as sick. If she had left my office with a confirmed illness diagnosis, her family would have been more comforted, as it would have validated what they already suspected. I found it very odd that they never considered her previous obesity as a sign of illness.

The World Health Organization (WHO) defines someone as overweight when they have a BMI > 25, and obese if their BMI is >30. A BMI of >40 is considered morbidly obese. BMI is calculated:

BMI = Weight (lbs) X 703 / Height^2 (in^2)

The CDC estimates that two-thirds of Americans are either overweight or obese. A full 33% of adults in the U.S. are considered obese, as are 20% of children, age 6-19. The majority of our citizens are either overweight or obese, and we think that is normal! According to international data collected in 2003, the U.S. is number one in the world in its prevalence of obesity.2 At that time, the prevalence of obesity in the U.S. was 30.6%. Mexico, which was second to the United States, was more than six percentage points lower for obesity, at 24%. Only one state in the U.S. had a rate of obesity less than 20%, and that was Colorado. Simply put, we are a fat nation. Being overweight or obese comes with a number of serious health conditions, including but not limited to the following:

- Coronary heart disease
- Type 2 diabetes
- Cancer
- Hypertension
- High cholesterol
- Stroke
- Liver and gallbladder disease
- Sleep apnea and respiratory problems
- Arthritis
- Gynecological problems, such as infertility and abnormal menses

Besides the health risks, obesity is also quite costly. Obesity related health care costs were estimated at $117 billion in the year 2000. Between 1987 and 2001, diseases associated with obesity accounted for 27% of the overall increase in medical costs. Medical expenditures for obese workers, depending on the severity of obesity and gender are estimated to be between 29% and 117% greater than expenditures for workers with normal weight.3 The obesity epidemic has grown steadily since 1980. The CDC estimates that the obesity rates for adults have doubled since that time, and for children it has tripled. We are fast becoming a super-sized nation, as we eat ourselves toward greater and greater incidences of obesity.

Diabetes

Another chronic condition plaguing our country is diabetes. Diabetes is a condition where the body does not make adequate amounts of insulin, or the body does not respond to the amount of insulin that is made. Insulin is a hormone that allows cells to consume glucose from the blood. Without insulin, glucose is not taken up into the body's tissue cells adequately and stays in the bloodstream, causing the body to suffer numerous metabolic conditions.

Diabetes comes in two forms of disease—type 1 and type 2. Although the mechanism of type 1 is not fully understood, it has classically been considered an immune complex disorder, triggered by some foreign agent, such as a viral infection. There is also considerable evidence in research literature that suggests the consumption of cow's milk may predispose some individuals to type 1 diabetes. In either case, type 1 diabetes is considered caused by an autoimmune process, a condition where the body's immune system attacks itself. Type 1 diabetes is considered rare, occurring in just 5-10% of all diabetics.4

The typical way type 1 diabetes is discovered is when an infant or a child as old as a young adolescent, has an episode of extremely elevated blood sugar, following an apparent viral syndrome. Frequently the child will experience a condition known as diabetic ketoacidosis that will require them to be hospitalized, and to receive an infusion of insulin to control their blood sugar and blood acid levels. Essentially, what happens is that insulin producing cells of the pancreas are destroyed, and the pancreas is no longer able to make insulin. An individual with this form of diabetes is truly insulin dependent, typically requiring multiple daily injections of the insulin hormone. This condition is also referred to as childhood or juvenile diabetes.

Type 2 diabetes, on the other hand, develops in a normally functioning pancreas, at least initially. Long before an individual meets the clinical definition of diabetes, they will go through a prolonged period of insulin resistance. In this state, the pancreas will produce ever increasing amounts of insulin, which is necessary to maintain a normal blood sugar level. Eventually the body becomes overwhelmed, and the pancreas can no longer produce enough insulin to consume the higher levels of glucose in the blood. The body loses the battle and blood sugar levels begin to rise. Our bodies fight the good fight and try desperately to alert us to what is going on. We will start to exhibit a condition, often referred to as pre-diabetes or insulin resistance, in many cases years or even decades prior to meeting the clinical criteria for type 2 diabetes. Are we paying attention?

Diabetes is associated with a number of significant medical problems. These include:

- Heart disease and stroke
- Blindness
- Kidney failure
- Peripheral artery disease (potentially resulting in amputation)
- Neurological disease, specifically peripheral neuropathy

In the case of type 2 diabetes, we have long known that controlling blood sugar has little if any impact on the progression of long-term diabetes complications such as blindness, heart disease, kidney failure, and peripheral arterial disease. Although Americans have unfortunately become accustomed to their increasing girth, they still seem to retain a healthy respect for the potential negative impact of diabetes.

I was once interviewed by a local TV news station on the topic of sudden cardiac death in young athletes. The news anchor and camera operator came to my office to perform the interview. While waiting for me to return to my office, they apparently entered into a discussion with one of my staff regarding our approach to treating heart disease and other chronic illnesses with nutritional intervention. After performing the interview with me on sudden cardiac arrest, the news anchor asked if she could come back and interview me on our approach to disease intervention using nutrition. She wanted to focus on the issue of heart disease and diabetes. She returned two months later and performed an extensive interview in my office.

Two of our patients who had gone through our program were also interviewed. The resulting story was aired locally. When the story aired, both the news station and my office received an overwhelming response in terms of phone calls and internet responses. My office received hundreds of calls on the diabetes story, compared to only one or two for the cardiac arrest story. The general public seems to have a much greater sense of concern about type 2 diabetes than sudden cardiac arrest!

What is the reason for such a different response? I believe it is because an individual whether they are personally dealing with a chronic condition like diabetes, or watching a loved one go through it, along with family members and friends, recognize the daily human struggle brought on by diabetes. There are daily challenges required in a diabetic's life because of the many complications associated with their disease. Their condition is never fully out of mind, thanks to constant reminders that come with daily medications, which may include insulin injections, and daily finger pricks to check blood glucose levels. The diabetic may also suffer more advanced disease states that exist in addition to their primary diabetes condition. They may be subject to heart attacks, stroke, blindness, kidney failure, or amputation. These added conditions only increase the burden of loved ones caring for them, with frequent doctor visits, hospitalizations, dialyses visits, and the like.

Such a lifestyle of prolonged and sustained sickness sharpens the awareness of how this disease affects not only themselves, but also their immediate family members and friends.

Arthritis
Despite running an active cardiology practice, the number one complaint I receive from all of my patients, collectively, relates to arthritis. These complaints run from neck, shoulder, elbow, knee, lower back, and hip pain. Patients complain regularly about joint aches and swelling. What are the facts about arthritis?[5]

- Approximately 46 million adults in the U.S. report being told by a doctor that they have some form of arthritis.
- Approximately 21% of adults in the U.S. report having a doctor diagnose them with arthritis.
- An estimated 67 million aged 18 years or older are projected to have a doctor diagnose arthritis by the year 2030.
- Two thirds of the people who have had a doctor diagnose arthritis are under the age of 65.
- It is estimated in the year 2003, arthritis and rheumatic conditions cost the U.S. economy $128 billion.
- Arthritis is the second most frequently reported chronic condition in the U.S.

Arthritis is primarily a condition caused by inflammation of the musculoskeletal hard and soft tissue (bones, joints, and muscles). In most, if not all, cases, it is considered an autoimmune complex disorder. Like many other chronic illnesses, there seems to be an increasing prevalence among the young with arthritis.

Other Chronic Illnesses

Although an exhaustive discussion of chronic illnesses is beyond the scope of this book, it is necessary to make mention of the fact that many other illnesses come under the classification of chronic illnesses, and collectively have a major impact on Americans. Examples include conditions such as dementia, gastrointestinal disorders, chronic fatigue disorders, chronic headache syndromes, and the like.

Additionally, chronic illnesses are rarely experiences in isolation but rather coexist with multiple other disorders. For instance, an individual who is obese often suffers from diabetes, and similarly an individual with diabetes often suffers from heart disease and high levels of cholesterol, as well as arthritis. I am seeing an increasing number of young people in my practice, who are coming to me with multiple chronic disorders. Many of these individuals will have arthritic syndromes, which may be one of a number of classes of inflammatory conditions such as lupus, rheumatoid arthritis, as well as heart disease, hypertension, and obesity.

The coexistence of such chronic disorders frequently leads to the use of multiple medications of different types and different classes. We often refer to this as polypharmacy, 'poly' being much or many, and 'pharmacy' being related to medications. Hence, the presence of multiple chronic disorders, along with the use of multiple medications with various side effects and drug-to-drug interactions, frequently leads to more illness, and in many cases, a faster decline in health and wellness. In dealing with any chronic illness, we can look at it from the perspective of a specific medical diagnosis or as an abnormal physiological condition of the human body. This is an important distinction, because if we just look at the illness as a defined medical diagnosis that may have been arrived at arbitrarily, we may miss an even more important condition.

For example, the diagnosis of diabetes requires, among other things, an elevated fasting blood sugar level. However, we know that diabetes is an abnormal physiological condition that is associated with heart, kidney, eye, and peripheral circulation disease. It is this abnormal physiological condition that causes diabetics to acquire these other problems and this condition begins long before the individual has an elevated fasting blood sugar.

The underlying physiological condition will progress for many years without a clinical diagnosis, causing early damage to the heart, eyes, kidneys, or peripheral circulation. By the time the individual has an elevated fasting blood glucose level, and receives a diabetes diagnosis, they may possibly have already contracted significant heart, kidney, or eye disease. This is an important consideration because when doctors treat patients medically, we typically treat them based on their clinical diagnosis. This may result in our treating just an outward manifestation of an underlying problem and not the problem itself.

Referring to our diabetes example again, we often treat fasting blood sugar levels. However, diabetes is not primarily a blood sugar disease, but one of abnormal cellular metabolism, among other things. Metabolism is the process of breaking down old cells and tissue parts and building new ones. When errors in metabolism occur, disease states can develop. Hence, heart disease, kidney disease, diabetes, and other chronic illnesses are rooted in abnormal metabolism. So, when we treat diabetes to improve blood sugar levels, we are having no effect on the underlying condition, and may possibly introduce unexpected side effects. In other words, the treatment can sometimes be worse than the disease.

"But doc, I'm going to die of something!"
When dealing with chronic illnesses, we in medicine often are focused on the potential impact of a particular disease, or set of diseases, on someone's mortality. This is especially true with chronic conditions of heart disease and cancer, as these are also the top two causes of death for Americans. As a result, a lot of attention is given to decreasing mortality rates caused by those diseases.

I frequently find the need to point out for my patients that although these conditions can shorten their lifespan, the greater immediate impact they will feel is from an impaired quality of life. People need to realize that the major benefit of preventing or reversing a chronic illness is the benefit of adding more life to their years, as opposed to more years to their life.

Bolder patients might argue they will die anyway, which is when I respond that all research supports the conclusion that the mortality rate of human beings is 100%, one death per person. None of us escapes this consequence. Ultimately, the quality of our days is what is most important.

I hope it is clear that the major impact of chronic illnesses is not only a shortened lifespan, but also a reduced quality of life. We must also be clear that a lower quality of life is not only felt by the individual suffering with a chronic illness, but also has a devastating effect on the lives of the loved ones around them. This is why we need to pursue aggressively the prevention, control, and reversal of chronic disease states—to provide a better way of life for all concerned. The key to these life-giving changes are already within our control.

෴

Chapter Three
Your Digestive System Owner's Manual

The study of the human body is very complex. It requires a lifetime of study to gain a good appreciation of everything that goes on. However, it is critical for all of us to have at least a basic understanding of how the body functions to recognize the impacts of nutritional choices on the health and sustainability of our body. This knowledge is what I hope provides the encouragement necessary for people to take control of their own health, knowing the consequences of not making better choices.

We all make this effort when it comes to our cars and appliances to get the best performance for our investment. Surely, our own bodies deserve the same basic understanding. For the sake of our health, we need to understand at least the basics of human biochemistry and physiology. This will help show the connection between proper nutrition and optimal body function.

To start, we need a few terms defined:
- Anatomy—Refers to the study of body structures, and the relationships among structures.
- Physiology—Deals with the function of body parts and body organ systems.
- Biochemistry—Includes the concept of chemical substances and their properties, and reactions within a living organism. The term biochemistry is a composite of two words, bio and chemistry. Chemistry is the composition of substances and their properties, and reactions with one another. Bio refers to life.

As we continue a discussion on how the body works, biochemistry will be a focus. Specifically, we will be referring to how chemical substances create structure and form, and how these chemical substances have properties that result in certain reactions between one another.

We will also talk about anatomy in terms of how the body is constructed, and about physiology in terms of how various body parts and organ systems function and interact with each other.

So, how are we put together? It's best to think of our bodies as levels of structural organization.₁ Like any other physical substance, the human body is made up of atoms, which are put together to form molecules. Molecules will subsequently form cellular structures. It is at the cellular level that living organisms are differentiated from non-living organisms. Hence, the basic unit of life for human beings is the human cell. When we think of molecules, there are two fundamental characteristics important for this discussion:

- They have chemical properties as discussed earlier, in the sense that they can react with each other to create different substances.
- They also have form and structure, which serve as building blocks or structural components of the human body.

As molecules come together to form cells, these cells become alike, taking on the same properties. Each has the ability to carry out chemical reactions, as well as to compose a specific form and structure. For example, a blood vessel has the structure and shape of a pipe. Blood vessels are each composed of cells, which are in turn composed of molecules.

Not only do blood vessels have the form and structure of a pipe, they are also able to constrict (become narrower), and dilate (become more open). These changes can be caused by nerves, hormones, or other chemical substances created by the body. Therefore, unlike a structural pipe in our bathroom plumbing—having a fixed shape, form, and length—a "pipe" in the human body can dilate or constrict when necessary. In addition, blood vessels in some parts of the body can constrict while others dilate, allowing for selective blood flow to areas of greater need or importance.

An example of this occurs when an individual bleeds excessively and suffers from shock. The body will shunt (transfer) blood to the most vital organs, such as the brain and the heart. This is just one example of how fearfully and wonderfully made our bodies are, with the ability to take on selective form and structure, based on physiologic needs.

As we look deeper into structural organization, we realize that cells come together to form tissue. Tissues are groups of similar cells that work together to carry out a uniform function within the body. Tissues are what come together to form an organ. At the organ level, structures are composed of two or more different types of tissue that carry out a specific function, or set of functions, within the body. Beyond the level of individual organs are systems. One or more organs come together to work in synchrony, carrying out a number of different functions and meeting various needs of the body.

Finally, we have the organizational level that is the human body itself, or the organism. All of the different organ systems come together to form the body, and these organ systems interact with one another to carry out the body's functions to live, grow, heal, and more.

Transforming Food into Body Energy

The gastrointestinal (GI) system is a synchronous group of organs that work together to extract nutrients the body needs from the foods we eat. Like other systems in the body, the GI system is lined with various different types of cells. There are mucous cells, parietal cells, and zymogenic cells. The technical names of these cells are not important. What is important is that these cells are structural in nature, creating the lining of the gastrointestinal tract and giving the intestines and the stomach distinct forms.

Beyond structural properties, these cells have chemical properties that allow organs like the stomach to carry out the important functions of digestion. This means that the stomach, for example, is not only a cavity or a structure where food is stored, but also an organ that carries out chemical reactions for digestion. Let's meet the major players in the digestion process, and see how nutrients from food are made available for our bodies to use. Digestion is a very complex process. For the purpose of this discussion, we can think of digestion as a process of breaking down food to extract needed nutrients and eliminating waste (i.e. cleansing).

Stomach

The process of digestion begins in the mouth as soon as we eat or drink something. Our mouth or oral cavity is connected to the esophagus and then to the stomach. The stomach's job is two-fold—food storage and digestion. Important nutrients are extracted for the body's use, while waste is accumulated for elimination. This activity is accomplished by breaking down the food we eat into smaller structural components, in part from the release of gastric (stomach) acid.

Small and Large Intestines

The organ structures of the small and large intestine work in conjunction with the stomach to carry out various digestive properties. When we eat, the stomach begins the process of breaking food down with secreted stomach acid. This creates gastric juices and acid that flows through sections of small intestine called the duodenum, the ileum, and then the jejunum to further break down the food. The ileum (the second part of the small intestines) contains a very large surface area. Stretched out, it would cover the surface area of a tennis court. Having a large surface area is important, as it allows the body to absorb more nutrients.

The small intestine receives help in the form of secretions from the liver and pancreas, through the duodenum, using bile ducts. These secretions help extract nutrients from food that the body needs, such as fat, protein, minerals, and vitamins. These nutrients are subsequently absorbed or transported into the bloodstream over the vast surface area of the middle segment of the small intestine, called the ileum.

The large intestine is an organ about 1.5m (4.9ft) in length, and is comprised of the cecum, colon, rectum, and anus. Its role is to pass solid waste material out of the body. This is the body's last opportunity to extract water from digested food. The more dehydrated the body is, the more water the body will extract from the digested remains within the large intestine.

If the body is well hydrated, the colon will absorb less water, and the solid remains in the colon will have a more liquid consistency, and be able to pass more easily through the colon and out the rectum. Conversely, solid remains will have a dryer consistency if the body is poorly hydrated, and pass more slowly through the colon, contributing to constipation.

Moreover, it is important to understand that the perfect stool should not be solid. It should be loose, semi-formed, and break up as we flush the toilet. If stools stay solid within the swirling water when the toilet is flushed, keeping their shape, this is a sign that your body may be dehydrated. Drinking water is a good way to hydrate yourself, but eating a variety of fruits and vegetables is even better. Hydrating yourself naturally with "plant-derived" water gives you the advantage of consuming water that is balanced with natural vitamins, protein, carbohydrates, and other nutrients. It also helps to alkalinize your bloodstream.

Liver

Another part of the GI system is the liver, which is a very, very important organ. It sits above the kidney on the right. The liver is a very complex structure that performs several key functions, including bile production to aid in digestion, and creating plasma proteins and cholesterol.

We usually think of cholesterol as bad, but that has to do with excess amounts of cholesterol that is found in our bloodstream. Cholesterol already exists in our bodies, naturally, and has beneficial functions. It lines the wall of every cell in our bodies and creates a protective coat around our peripheral nerves. It is also responsible for the production of testosterone, estrogen, and cortisone hormones. In addition, cholesterol helps to form components of bile salts and vitamin D in the skin.

Here is an overview of the major functions of the liver:
- **Carbohydrate Metabolism**—The liver converts glucose to glycogen, which is the storage form of sugar when blood sugar is high, and converts glycogen back to glucose (releasing sugar from storage) when blood sugar is low. The liver can convert other sugars and amino acids to glucose if needed, as well as convert glucose to fats.

- **Fat Metabolism**—The liver breaks down fat molecules and creates other molecules that transport fat, cholesterol, and fatty acids within the body. Cholesterol is broken down into bile salts, and used in the intestines for the absorption of fats, cholesterol, phospholipids, etc. The liver will also store fat that is not immediately needed.

- **Protein Metabolism**—The liver is where ammonia is removed from amino acids so they can be converted to carbohydrates or fats. Ammonia, which is a toxic substance, is converted to urea and excreted in the urine. The liver also produces proteins for the body (albumin, prothrombin, etc.) and develops molecules to prevent blood clotting (heparin).

- **Removal of Drugs and Hormones**—The liver plays an important role in removing harmful substances from our bodies. It can excrete or detoxify antibiotics, and alter or excrete steroid hormones.

- **Excretion of Bile**—Bilirubin from worn out blood cells is absorbed by the liver and excreted in the bile. From there, the bilirubin can be further broken down in the intestines and excreted in the feces.

- **Storage**—The liver stores vitamins A, B12, D, E, and K, as well as iron and copper minerals.

- **Cleansing the Blood**—Worn-out red and white blood cells, along with some bacteria that may have entered the bloodstream, get removed by the liver.

- **Vitamin D Activation**—The liver takes Vitamin D released from the skin or intestines and converts it into its more active form.

Pancreas

The pancreas is a small organ about six inches long, located in the upper abdomen, next to the small intestine. Its role in digestion is to complete the job of breaking down proteins, carbohydrates, and fats using a combination of secretions from the pancreas, as well as from the intestines. The pancreas is also part of the body's endocrine system, secreting a hormone called insulin, which aid in digestion by adjusting sugar levels in the blood. Insulin accomplishes this task by sending signals to the cells to use glucose extracted from the foods we eat.

Kidneys and Urinary System

Our bodies have two kidneys, with one on the right side of our bodies and one on the left. The right kidney sits slightly below the left kidney because the liver is positioned above it on that side. Blood flows into the kidney through the renal (kidney) artery, is filtered, and then exits through the renal vein. Around 190 liters of blood flows through our kidneys every day. At about 25% of our total circulation, that is a lot of blood!

Here is an overview of what the kidneys do for the body:

*   **Blood filtration**—The kidneys filter the blood flowing through them to remove substances the body does not need, such as medications, by-products of normal metabolism, and food additives.

*   **Electrolyte balancing**—The kidneys, at the same time, work to balance our electrolytes, controlling the levels of potassium, sodium, and other electrolytes, such as phosphorus, magnesium, and calcium in our blood. Electrolytes have to be regulated. If potassium levels in your blood are too high, you can go into cardiac arrest. If potassium levels are too low, you can go into cardiac arrest. You may eat ten bananas in a single day, which would bombard your system with potassium. Fortunately, your kidneys "have your back," as they say. If they are operating normally, your kidneys will make sure your blood retains just the right amount of potassium, while filtering out the excess.

*   **Water regulation**—Our bodies are about 75% water, and yes, it is possible to over-hydrate yourself. When you drink water, your thirst mechanism is supposed to shut off and tell you to stop drinking. Your thirst goes away. However, we have all heard stories of people who have drunk excessive amounts of water because of a bet. When someone over-hydrates, they experience water toxicity. This is because their body is not able to

regulate fast enough. Under a normal situation, the kidneys control the right amount of water needed for proper hydration. When we become dehydrated, our kidneys are not able to function at their optimal level. The blood flow into the kidneys becomes less, which results in less filtration. Less filtration leads to keeping more unneeded and dangerous substances floating around inside of our bodies. This can lead to illness. That is why we hear so much about the importance of staying hydrated. How do you know if you are dehydrated? While there is no specific test, people will generally experience symptoms such as feeling weak, tired, having dry skin, and consistently dark urine. These are indicators of dehydration. Some people also have headaches, are constipated, have dry mouth, or just feel thirsty.

- **Urine production**—All of the fluid filtered out of the blood by the kidneys flows through the ureters, into the bladder, and finally out the urethra as urine. The remaining blood then flows out of the kidneys through the renal vein, into the inferior vena cava, and back to the heart.

Summary

My goal is for every person to have a basic understanding of how their body functions to help them recognize how their nutritional choices impact their health and overall quality of life. My hope is that once people are educated about the consequences of their decisions, they can make the right choices. Our bodies are structural in nature, made up of cells that come together to form tissues. Tissues come together to form organs, which work together within the body to carry out functions related to living, growing, healing, and more. The gastro-intestinal (GI) system is a group of structures that effectively works together to break down food, extract needed nutrients, and eliminate waste and toxins.

The GI system is superbly designed to perform these functions; however, our food choices can wind up bombarding the system to such a degree that it cannot keep up with the demands for filtering and breaking down substances the body does not need. When this occurs, waste and toxins cannot be properly eliminated from our bodies. As these byproducts accumulate, it leads to chronic or even acute disease states. Now that we know how our body works to process the foods we eat, let's look at some nutritional basics, to see how we can optimally fuel our body.

෬

Chapter Four
The Truth About Good Nutrition

Nearly 100% of my patients and wellness clients agree in theory that following a diet based on good nutrition is important and has a significant influence over their health and well-being. Unfortunately, too many do not recognize what a nutritionally sound diet consists of. They have bought into the ageless perception that anything taken in moderation is okay. As a cardiologist, I know that moderation is inadequate at best, and potentially even deadly.

Furthermore, achieving optimal nutrition goes beyond keeping track of calories, protein, fats, carbohydrates, and portion sizes. Although these are important aspects of how we nourish our bodies, our nutritional health is based on factors that are more fundamental. In the previous chapter, we talked about how complex the human body is. We now understand it in the context of its general anatomy, physiology, and biochemistry. The body is a very complex structure of anatomical, biochemical, and physiological organ systems. The intricacies of how these systems function and interact with each other are beyond our full understanding. However, the most important concept is how the function of these organ systems is heavily influenced by the food we eat.

Food, by definition, is a material substance that consists of essential body nutrients. These nutrients are commonly known as carbohydrates, fats, proteins, vitamins, water, phytonutrients, and minerals. They are ingested and assimilated by the body to produce energy, stimulate growth, and carry out many other functions to maintain life. Nutrients have various chemical properties. Some are mostly structural in nature, while others are more functional.

There are seven known types of nutrients:
- Carbohydrates
- Fats

- Proteins
- Minerals
- Vitamins
- Water
- Phytonutrients

Carbohydrates, proteins, and lipids are digested by protein structures, known as enzymes. This primarily occurs in the gastrointestinal tract. The end product of these molecular compounds as they reach our cells in their various molecular types form the building blocks of different body parts. Although we commonly think of nutritional substances as sources of energy, they serve a large variety of other needs for the body.

Carbohydrates are the primary energy source for the human body; however, fats and proteins can also be used for energy. Amino acids on the other hand are structural in nature and the building blocks of protein that exist in various tissues, cells, and organs. Other types of nutrients such as vitamins, minerals, and phytonutrients allow the body to facilitate numerous other complex functions such as DNA repair, cell regeneration, immune system maintenance, and much more.

What is important to understand is that food consists of a variety of complex chemical substances that the body utilizes to maintain its structural integrity, as well as its delicate biochemical and physiological balances.

Therefore, nutrients must have similar basic properties as the human body itself, and these properties must be complementary to the body.

The Battle for Nutritional Excellence

It is difficult to ignore the fact that our standard American diet is making us sick, and even killing us, one bite at a time. Our food consists of substances that are either inherently bad nutrients or substances that have been altered or processed in such a way that they are transformed into toxins.

The vast majority of illnesses we suffer from are simply side effects of the bad food we eat. Arthritis (gouty arthritis)[1], heart disease[2], high cholesterol3, depression4, and more are the results of biochemical reactions of the food we eat that cause adverse conditions in our bodies.

So, why does the body need nourishment anyway? If in fact, the body has all of the basic molecules and structures it needs from the beginning, why are these molecular structures not capable of simply maintaining themselves?

We have to consider that the body is subjected to wear and tear through external conditions. This can be the result of variations in temperature, daily use (or abuse), or through our process of growing as human beings from youth to adulthood. The process of living subjects the body to ongoing wear and tear, requiring constant repair. This ongoing rebuilding and repairing is necessary for the processes of growth, development, and health maintenance.

> The vast majority of illnesses we suffer
> from are simply side effects of the bad
> food we eat.

A good analogy would be to compare what our bodies require for optimal performance to that of our car or perhaps our home. These things might start out as new, but through the process of "wear and tear" they require regular maintenance. The wood on a house over time has to be repainted. The tires on the car have to be changed, as does the oil. As oil passes through the compartments of the engine, it is exposed to buildups of sediment and dirt, and other types of particulate matter that are not good for the engine. In the same way that an automobile or house structure needs to be improved, rebuilt, and remodeled, the body has to undergo a similar process.

The body is designed to perform its own rebuilding and repairing when properly nourished. For example, we know both the skin and intestinal lining are replaced over certain periods of time. So in order to carry out this process of rebuilding and maintaining itself, the body has to be nourished properly. That is why *how* we nourish our bodies is important. That is to say, the quality of nutrition put into the body has a direct impact on the quality of the body's components that are rebuilt. This is why the old saying, "You are what you eat," is quite accurate. In fact, the statement "you are what you eat" originates back to the early and mid 1800s.

A French writer by the name of Anthelme Brillat-Savarin wrote in 1826, "Tell me what you eat, and I will tell you what you are." (English translation from the original French). In 1863 and 1864, Ludwig Andreas Feuerbach wrote, "Man is what he eats." (English translation).s Both of these men intended for their quotations to be taken literally. They were stating that what we eat has an absolute bearing on one's state of mind and health. Hence it has been known for centuries that good nutrition is directly related to good health, and conversely, poor nutrition is related to poor health.

The Opposite of Good Nutrition—Poison

We must consider that the antithesis of good nutrition is poison! The definition of poison is that of a substance with an inherent tendency to destroy life or impair health. We often think of a poisonous substance as something that leads to immediate death, a violent reaction, or an acute, severe illness when consumed.

> We must consider that the antithesis of good nutrition is poison!

However, any substance that has the ability to impair health, at any level and to any degree, by definition can be considered a poison. In contrast, most nutrients that are beneficial for the body do not have the inherent ability to impair health, but rather have the important qualities of enhancing health—even when consumed in large amounts.

So, which foods are good for us, and which foods are bad?

Identifying Foods as Good or Bad

It is important to understand foods in terms of classifications. The best way to classify foods is based on their origin—plant-based foods or animal-based foods. This raises two important questions. First, is plant consumption essential to the nourishment of humans? Secondly, is animal consumption essential to the nourishment of humans? To answer these questions we simply have to consider how organisms from the animal or plant kingdoms are nourished. Plants, as you know, primarily receive their nourishment from inorganic sources. Specifically, these sources include some form of soil, water, carbon dioxide, and sunlight. Of note, pollination usually occurs with the assistance of bees, which are non-plant life forms. However, this is a reproductive process and can occur without bees. Nevertheless, plant life utilizes soil (and its associated minerals), carbon dioxide, water, and sunlight for its nourishment.

Organisms from the animal kingdom on the other hand, rely on organic and inorganic sources for their nourishment. Primary sources of nourishment for animals are oxygen, water, sunlight, and plants. Carnivorous animals indirectly rely on plants because the animals they eat are usually plant eaters, or prey upon plant-eating animals. Green plants go through a process known as photosynthesis, allowing them to create sugars from energy generated directly from sunlight. Plants can grow, nourish, and replenish themselves with adequate sources of soil, water, carbon dioxide, and sunlight. Animals, specifically humans, require plants, oxygen, water, and sunlight for nourishment. Plants provide humans with an abundant source of vitamins, minerals, carbohydrates, fats, protein, phytonutrients, and water for nourishment. In fact, when consumed in adequate amounts, plants can theoretically provide humans with all of their nutritional needs other than sunlight. Although most Americans consume large amounts of animal products as part of their nourishment, considerable scientific evidence shows that individuals who exclude animal food sources from their diets are generally healthier.[6]

Two critical questions must be addressed:
1. Do human beings need animal based foods along with plant based foods for their nourishment?
2. Is it important for foods to be eaten as close to their natural state as possible? Moreover, do foods become less nourishing when they are processed more?

Is There A Human Need for Animal-Based Food?

Epidemiological data strongly shows that individuals can live on diets consisting of plant-based foods alone.[7] Furthermore, scientific studies have strongly indicated that individuals who live either solely or predominantly on plant based diets are actually healthier than individuals who live on mostly animal flesh diets.[8] Much media attention has been given to the pursuit of low-carb diets. Two studies were done to track the long-term impact of low-carb diets. A total of close to 130,000 adults, ranging in age from 34 to 75 were tracked for an average of 23 years. Participants all ate low-carb diets, with some choosing animal-based sources of protein and fat, while others chose vegetable based sources of these same nutrients. None who participated in the study started with any clinical evidence of heart disease, cancer, or diabetes. The results showed that those who chose animal-based low-carb diets had higher mortality from all causes than those participants who chose vegetable-based low-carb diets. This was true for both men and women participants in these studies.[9]

Dr. T. Colin Campbell, author of *The China Study*,[10] clearly defines the importance of plant-based nutrition over animal-based nutrition. There is strong scientific evidence showing associations with chronic diseases, such as an increase in cholesterol [11], elevation of blood pressure [12], osteoporosis, and type 2 diabetes with the consumption of animal flesh in any form, whether it is beef, chicken, turkey, or even fish.[13]

This evidence strongly supports the superiority of plant-based foods over animal based foods with regard to maintaining human health. Furthermore, this evidence shows that animal-based foods are associated with disease states linked to the impairment of health. Hence, not only are animal-based foods less healthy, they are much more detrimental. If you remember the definition of poison presented earlier, we can now see how the consumption of animal-based foods could be considered poisonous to our bodies. The scientific evidence supports the notion of plant based foods being superior to animal-based foods for human health.

Are Unprocessed Plant Foods Better than Processed Plant Foods?

Does it really matter what condition the plant food is in when consumed? This question may be more difficult to address. Although most of our scientific data deals with epidemiological or observational studies related to the consumption of plant-based versus animal based foods, we do not have a clear delineation of how these plant-based foods were prepared for the most part. We have, however, some scientific data and evidence showing the importance of how foods are processed, and the ability of certain methods to diminish a food's nutritional value.

There is significant evidence that when vegetables are cooked, they lose some of their nutritional value.[14] We know when vegetables are deep-fried or battered they will have a higher fat content, and as a result, be associated with adverse health conditions. We can take the freshest, most nutrient-dense, organically grown vegetables available and boil them to death, and end up pouring what our body needs for good health right down the drain. Alternatively, we can batter and deep-fry those same vegetables, and they become toxic to our system.[15] Fried foods are linked to adverse health conditions, like obesity, diabetes, and heart disease. Additionally, studies show that there is a correlation between the amount of toxins that are developed in food as a result of temperature increases and how long the food is exposed to heat. Therefore, one does not have to fry food to make it more toxic. Grilling and baking at high temperatures can have the same detrimental effects. Microwave oven cooking has also been shown to have adverse effects on foods.[16]

Furthermore, we know that toxic substances such as acrylamide are not found in foods that are steamed or boiled at relatively short durations, or heated at low temperatures. Acrylamide is a chemical compound that forms naturally when a wide variety of foods are heated at high temperatures. This includes coffee, chocolate, almonds, French fries, potato chips, crackers, and even some fruits and vegetables.[17] Therefore, it is not too big of a leap to consider at the very least, over-processing of plant-based foods can be related to disease formation, and therefore, the less processing our foods go through the more valuable they are for ensuring good health.

We also need to understand where our food comes from. There is scientific evidence that organically grown vegetables have higher nutrient content than conventionally grown vegetables.[18] But there is more to the story. The conditions in which food substances are grown may very well also be important. Plant-based foods grown in poor soil conditions may be less optimal than plant-based foods grown in better conditions. Lettuce grown in poor soil, for example, can only absorb the nutrients available in that soil. Another concern, lettuce crops using chemicals for pest management will absorb those chemicals, and we, in-turn, ingest those chemicals when we eat a salad mixed with those greens.

Clearly, with less processing of foods, either during its development or its preparation is associated with higher nutritional value and possibly better health when consumed. However, there is evidence that some forms of processing, specifically raw juicing, may actually be beneficial.[19] Although little has been published in the mainstream peer reviewed scientific journals, books written by several naturopathic doctors have reported on the numerous benefits of raw fruit and vegetable juices for various medical conditions.[20] I can also speak from my own experience of these benefits, having observed numerous clinical benefits of raw juices in my patients with conditions such as coronary artery disease, congestive heart failure, arthritis, diabetes, hypertension, and many other chronic diseases. Based on the available data, it is reasonable to state that unprocessed or minimally processed foods are more beneficial than processed foods. Additionally, the greater the extent of the processing the less nutritious, or perhaps, more toxic the food is likely to be. We can summarize levels of processing in the following way.

Figure 4.1

Type of Processing	Potential Health Effects	Comments
Raw Juicing	++	The benefits of this form of processing may be due to the fact that the food is broken down in a way that the need to chew is minimized or eliminated. Also, the nutrients may be absorbed in an energy conservative manner.
Raw Blending (in the form of dairy free smoothies)	++	See comments for raw juicing
Whole raw food consumption	+ to ++	
Lightly Steamed or Boiled	+/- to +	The specifics of how the food is steamed or boiled and the type of food may determine whether it is neutral or beneficial
Moderately Steamed or Boiled	+/- to +	Dehydrating or very slow warming of foods that do not have a high fat content can be neutral. No browning should occur.
Dehydrated or Warmed or Baked at temperatures less than 200°F	+/-	
Dehydrated or Warmed, or Baked at temperatures greater than 200°F	- to +/-	If significant browning occurs, this could be detrimental.
Baking at temps greater than 300°F	-	Acrylamide formation usually occurs.
Grilled	- -	
Sautéed (Shallow Fried)	- -	Acrylamide formation usually occurs.
Microwaved	- -	
Deep Fried	- -	Acrylamide formation usually occurs.

++ very beneficial; + beneficial; +/- neutral; - detrimental; - - very detrimental

The Nutritional Sufficiency of a Plant-based Diet
I cannot be on a plant-based diet long-term. Where would I get my protein?

This is one of the most common complaints I hear when I explain to patients the superior nature of a plant-based diet. I find people hold a wrong perception that plants cannot supply all of the essential nutrients the body requires to function properly. This is sadly due in part to very successful lobbying by the meat and dairy industries to convince Americans they cannot be healthy without animal flesh, milk, and cheese in their diets. The American Dietetic Association (ADA) came out with the following proclamation in 2009: "It is the position of the American Dietetic Association that appropriately planned vegetarian diets, including total vegetarian or vegan diets, are healthful, nutritionally adequate, and may provide health benefits in the prevention and treatment of certain diseases. Well-planned vegetarian diets are appropriate for individuals during all stages of the life cycle, including pregnancy, lactation, infancy, childhood, adolescence, and for athletes."[21]

The ADA defines a vegetarian diet as one that does not include meat or seafood, or food products that contain meat or seafood. The results of their evidence-based review showed that those who follow a vegetarian diet have a lower risk of death from heart disease, they maintain lower cholesterol levels, have lower blood pressure, and have lower rates of hypertension and type 2 diabetes than nonvegetarians. This is likely because vegetarians tend to consume fewer foods containing saturated fats and cholesterol, while favoring fruits, vegetables, whole grains, nuts, soy products, fiber, and phytochemicals.

With regards to protein, the ADA states that when a variety of plant foods are consumed over the course of a day, the diet will provide all of the necessary amino acids, and ensure adequate nitrogen retention and use in healthy adults. This statement debunks the myth that vegetarians need to combine certain plant foods to create complete proteins at each meal. Even athletes, according to the ADA, can meet all of their protein requirements from a plant-based diet. Amino acids are the building blocks of protein, with eight specific amino acids considered critical, and therefore called essential amino acids. These cannot be manufactured by our bodies and therefore need to be supplied by the foods we eat. Concentrated sources of amino acids available in plants come from peas, beans, lentils, spinach, kale, quinoa, sprouted grains and many other sources.[22]

Everything a person needs nutritionally is found in plant-based foods, with a couple of exceptions in certain situations. Some people may find they need a B12 supplement to meet their particular needs. Vitamin B12 comes from bacteria and other single-celled organisms. It is a common belief that in days gone by, when our hygiene practices were less rigid than they are today, there were traces of B12 that were in the soil and on fruits and vegetables that would be consumed. There are also bacteria in the intestines of animals that create B12 and ends up in the meat.

In today's environment with more focus on cleanliness, people might not get enough B12 to meet their needs. Although, individuals who consume regular amounts of raw fermented vegetables may obtain adequate B12 from the live cultures in these foods. A good example is the ubiquitous nature of antibacterial soaps in today's environment.

With frequent use of antibacterial soaps for washing hands, we can avoid passing colds and germs, but we kill many "good" bacteria in the process too. So as it relates to the need or not for a B12 supplement, it's best to have your blood checked to make sure you are getting adequate amounts.

The other nutrient some people lack adequate supply of is Vitamin D. Technically, Vitamin D is not a vitamin, but rather a hormone produced by our skin when exposed to sunlight, and converted to its active form as it passes through our liver and kidneys. Our bodies use Vitamin D in its active form to aid calcium absorption and to help protect cells against cancer. It's a very important nutritional element for these reasons, especially for women who may be at greater risk for osteoporosis.

Unlike our ancestors, most of us don't get adequate exposure to sunlight, which is the best source of Vitamin D. Many more of us work in office environments and fail to get outside to take advantage of the healthy benefits of sunlight. If this is the case for you, I would first recommend that you try to get outside more often to take a brisk walk, exposed to the sun. With adequate sun exposure there's no need for additional Vitamin D supplementation, and it can do wonders for your overall health and sense of well-being. That's why I recommend this approach first. If this is not possible, you may need to take a Vitamin D supplement.

What about Calcium?

Questions are frequently raised about getting sufficient calcium with a plant-based diet. It is unfortunate that there is a common misperception that the only way to get adequate calcium in your diet is to drink milk and eat dairy products. This may be what the dairy industry wants us to believe, but the science is clear on this issue.[23] Dr. Fuhrman addresses this concern in his book *Eat to Live*.[24]

It is well established that plant-based foods are not only adequate sources of dietary calcium but are superior sources compared to animal sources, specifically dairy. The regular consumption of dairy and meat products results in urinary losses of calcium, as calcium is released from the bones to neutralize the acid load in the bloodstream caused by eating animal protein. This likely creates a negative balance of calcium intake and loss. Prolonged negative calcium balances could result in the development of osteoporosis. Therefore, if meats, dairy, and fish are eliminated from the diet in place of plant-based food, the body's need for overall calcium intake could be reduced. 25

Summary

Food by definition is a material substance that consists of essential body nutrients. These nutrients can be structural in nature and/ or functional in nature. The seven principal types of nutrients—carbohydrates, fats, proteins, minerals, vitamins, water, and phytonutrients— serve as either energy sources, structural building blocks, or catalysts (promoters) for important biological functions. They have similar basic properties as the human body itself, and these properties are ideally complementary to the body.

The problem is that we as Americans do not eat nutritionally excellent foods to a large degree. In fact, our standard American diet can be blamed for the poor health conditions that many of us face. The vast majority of our illnesses are the direct result of side effects brought on by the foods we eat. We must consider that the antithesis of good nutrition is poison! Any substance that has the ability to impair health, at any level and to any degree, by definition can be considered a poison. Therefore, we need to be clear on how the food choices we make impact the performance of our bodies.

There is significant scientific evidence that plant-based foods are superior to animal-based foods for human health. Furthermore, we know that how foods are originally grown and how they are processed, also affects how nutritious these foods are for our bodies to use efficiently. It is also clear from a recent position taken by the American Dietetic Association (ADA), regarding the nutritional adequacy of vegetarian and vegan diets, that momentum is building for a revolutionary change in the way we understand nutrition. The ADA is a very conservative organization by design and purpose. Their statements, along with the growing body of scientific evidence, may greatly contribute to a change in how the medical profession can educate and treat patients to improve their quality of life.

Chapter Five
How to Prevent, Control, & Reverse Chronic Diseases

In the United States, we spend approximately 16% of our gross domestic product on the treatment of disease, specifically on health care.[1] This is significantly more than other developed nations. We also do a poor job as a nation of preventing costly hospital admissions for chronic conditions, like asthma or complications from diabetes. Chronic diseases affect our ability to work and our day-to-day productivity, thus impacting our economic wellbeing. Chronic diseases affect our quality of social interaction. They also affect our emotional wellbeing, bringing about pain, suffering, sickness, and emotional distress. As a result, living with chronic disease creates a huge overall daily impact on our society, making it extremely important to learn not only how to control or reverse chronic diseases, but even better, how to prevent them.

Disease, by definition, is an impairment of health or a condition of abnormal function. When such a condition remains over a prolonged period of time in a persistent or intermittent state, it is considered a chronic disease. While the body has the means to maintain itself, the degree to which the body can repair or maintain itself is based on the quality of the nourishment we provide it from the foods we eat.

What does it mean to prevent, control, or reverse chronic diseases?

I recall being asked by one of my wellness clients if she had gotten rid of her diabetes after starting to eat only minimally processed plant based foods and achieving normal blood sugars. Other patients in my clinical practice ask if they can avoid developing the amount of heart disease their parents suffered from. These questions underscore the critical issue of differentiating between disease prevention, control, and reversal.

To prevent something means to stop it or hinder it from happening. To control something means to hold it in restraint or dominate it. Reversal is the act of turning something back or redirecting it. The difficulty with distinguishing between preventing, controlling, or reversing a disease state has more to do with understanding the nature of the particular disease rather than the above definitions. For example, a hypothetical 52-year-old woman with a family history of breast cancer decides to follow a healthy lifestyle, which includes eating a minimally processed plant-based diet, getting regular exercise, and routine exposure to sunlight. Prior to the start of this lifestyle change, she has 64 clinically undetectable breast cancer cells in her left breast, with a normal physical exam and mammogram. Twenty years later, after continuing with the lifestyle change without interruption, she has no evidence of breast cancer, by exam or on a mammogram.

Clinically, she started the lifestyle change without breast cancer, and continued to have no breast cancer twenty years later. Based on a clinical evaluation, we can only say that she "prevented" breast cancer. However, if we could take a microscopic look into her breast tissue before and after the twenty-year period, we would be able to say more. We could say that she reversed the cancer, if the 64 cells were reduced to none after twenty years, or that the breast cancer was controlled if the number of cancer cells were about the same.

Our ability to truly state whether we are preventing, controlling, or reversing disease depends on our ability to detect the state of that disease at distinct points in time. With disease states that are severe enough to measure with routine clinical tests and evaluations, we can clearly document findings that show a partial reversal or control of that disease state when nutritional intervention is used. In the case of prevention, it is much more difficult to determine in an absolute manner, because of the occult nature in which many disease states begin.

> *...a whole foods, plant-based diet can prevent disease states, such as cancer, heart disease, obesity, diabetes, cataracts, macular degeneration, Alzheimer's, cognitive dysfunction, multiple sclerosis, osteoporosis, and many other diseases. Furthermore, a plant-based diet can benefit people regardless of their genes or personal disposition.*

For practical purposes, we generally define disease prevention, control, or reversal in the context of our current ability to detect disease clinically. Control and reversal may co-exist, as is the case when an individual with heart failure achieves partial reversal of his heart failure with subsequent control of the disorder.

Preventing Disease

We know not all nutrients are created equal. For optimal nourishment to prevent disease, we need to provide the body with substances that contain nutrients similar to the basic components of the body. These substances will have both chemical and structural characteristics.

Some nutrients are superior, based on their inherent properties to provide completeness in what our bodies need. They are more nutritionally efficient and should represent our primary choices for foods we eat. We know from a substantial body of evidence from studies done all over the world that a whole foods, plant-based diet can prevent disease states, such as cancer, heart disease, obesity, diabetes, cataracts, macular degeneration, Alzheimer's, cognitive dysfunction, multiple sclerosis, osteoporosis, and many other diseases.

Furthermore a plant-based diet can benefit people regardless of his or her genes, or personal disposition. This makes consuming whole, plant based foods a superior diet, compared to consumption of animal-based foods, to support prevention of a majority of diseases.[2]

Nevertheless, achieving optimal nutrition goes beyond just consuming plant-based foods.

Equally important is the condition under which the plants are grown,[3] and the extent to which they are processed. These factors influence nutritional quality. Therefore, it is critical to understand that optimal nutrition consists of plant-based foods that are grown in optimal conditions, and minimally processed prior to consumption.

The degree to which the body can repair itself to an optimal level will determine its ability to function normally and maintain what is considered a healthy state. Therefore, we can say that the foundation of optimal human function lies in the body's ability to nourish itself. The foundation of disease prevention is also based in optimal nutrition. This is well understood, because many disease states have been associated with nutritional deficits of various types. We know that when individuals go without nutrition at all, they will succumb to severe illness and eventually death if nourishment is not provided. While any form of nutrition is sufficient for minimal, basic survival, the body requires the best form of nutrition to perform in its optimal state. This is why minimally processed, plant based nutrition is the best way to prevent disease.

Controlling Disease

Many diseases people suffer from are due to an impaired function of one or more body systems. This may have been caused by physical injury, physiological insult, or even insufficient nutrition. Most chronic diseases are progressive in nature, meaning they continue to get worse over time. For example, diabetes can progress in a fashion such that it will result in eye, kidney, or heart disease. Lupus can progress to affect the kidneys and lungs. Hence, controlling a disease state means preventing it from worsening and affecting other parts of the body.

Disease control often occurs in association with partial reversal of the disease state. In our patients with hypertension and diabetes, we observe that they achieve improvement in their blood pressure and fasting blood glucose when they follow a plant-based diet. However, their blood pressures and fasting blood glucose levels will worsen when they deviate from their nutritionally excellent program. This is an example of partial reversal and control of a disease state. The underlying pathophysiological process remains present, but exists in a dormant state. It can be "reactivated" if exposed to the right amount of nutritionally poor foods.

Reversing Disease

The demonstration of disease reversal is often done using disease markers as surrogates of the disease state. For example, because of the close association of blood cholesterol with heart disease, the reduction of cholesterol is often used as a marker for the reversal or partial reversal of heart disease. Similarly, blood pressure reduction, weight control, and improvement in heart function or kidney function can all be used as markers for at least partial disease reversal.

In some cases, we are able to correlate biochemical findings with disease states. Such is the case in a number of studies that looked at the correlation of insulin resistance with accumulation of fat inside muscle cells. Independent researchers have found a strong association between fat inside of muscle cells and insulin resistance. Subsequent studies have shown that eating a plant-based diet is associated with a decrease in the amount of fat inside muscle cells.[4]

Individuals who participate in our Nutritional Boot Camp program have shown significant reduction in blood pressure, C-reactive protein (a marker for inflammation), weight, and waistline size. We have also seen reductions in HgbA1c and cholesterol levels in as short a span as four weeks. Our findings are consistent with early and partial disease reversal and control.

In 1996, Dr. Caldwell Esselstyn impressively proved that plant-based nutrition has the ability to restore cardiac function, and to do it quickly.[5] He worked with a patient who demonstrated poor circulation to a portion of her heart muscle, predisposing her to the risk of a significant cardiac event. Within ten days of adopting a plant-based diet, along with a low dose of a cholesterol reducing drug, her cholesterol levels dropped from 248 mg/dL to 137. After just three weeks, he rescanned her heart and discovered restored circulation in the area of her heart that was previously compromised! Dr. Esselstyn discusses this patient in his book, *Prevent and Reverse Heart Disease*. He also discusses the results of another study, which was reported in the *New England Journal of Medicine*. That particular study by another research team did not provide the same positive outcome for patients that his study did. This intrigued him. By contacting the study's author, Dr. Esselstyn learned that while this other study was also focused on aggressively reducing cholesterol levels, the method involved massive doses of cholesterol-lowering drugs alone, *without* making any changes to the way people in the study ate. Esselstyn commented, "Despite profound cholesterol reduction with medication, the arterial plaque inflammation (the fire) and disease progression were inevitable because the patients were still ingesting the toxic American diet (the gasoline)." Rather than contra-dict his study, Esselstyn found the results of his other author's study reinforced his claims that the key to successful disease state reversal is in food choices, and not in prescribing drugs alone to artificially and temporarily affect the disease state.

In many cases, disease is brought about, or perhaps accelerated, by poor nutrition. While natural biochemical substances from unprocessed plant-based foods are beneficial, artificial substances from processed foods can e harmful. A western diet that consists of heavily processed foods and predominantly animal flesh foods (including eggs and dairy) is widely accepted to predispose people to most of the chronic ill-nesses that plague our society. In this situation, we must understand it is not so much the lack of optimal nutrition having the effect, as it is the excess of suboptimal nutrition. Of particular concern are foods that directly result in making us sicker and therefore can be classified as toxic or even poisonous.

The first step in using nutrition as a form of therapy to reverse dis-ease is to remove all suboptimal nutrition that has had a direct impact on our health. By removing foods that are toxic from our diet, we bring about the first phase of healing. The body is allowed to reverse its condition when the offending agents are removed. The removal of substances such as processed animal products (chicken, fish, turkey, beef, pork, all wild game, eggs, milk, cheese, and all other foods contain-ing non-human animal milk), processed carbohydrates, and processed sugars allows the body to remove toxic waste substances that are the byproducts of metabolizing these suboptimal foods. This allows the body to cleanse itself.

Once we eliminate foods that are harmful to our body, we allow it to start rebuilding itself in a way that restores its ability to carry out physiological functions in an optimal manner. Furthermore, by introducing minimally processed, natural plant-based foods, we further enhance the rebuilding process. Simply stated, optimal foods beget optimal health.

> *Of particular concern are foods that directly result in making us sicker and therefore can be classified as toxic or even poisonous.*

Although the complete concept of disease states and disease development is far beyond the scope of this book, suffice it to say that the body has an inherent ability to repair itself, and can prevent, control, and reverse disease when nourished properly. However, the effort required by the body to reverse disease exceeds what is needed to maintain health alone. That is why nutritional excellence is especially important when there is a disease present that needs to be overcome.

The Nutrition Controversy

> *Let your food be your medicine and your medicine your food.*
> **—Hippocrates**

Despite a mountain of scientific evidence proving a positive connection between eating animal flesh and animal byproducts to the development of heart disease, stroke, hypertension, diabetes, osteoporosis, and prostate cancer, the USDA continues to promote meat and dairy as key components of a balanced diet. This could be due to pressure from industry lobbyists shaping their recommendations that are then sold to a trusting public. In 1991, Dr. Esselstyn assembled a blue-ribbon panel of leading scientists, nationally recognized for their expertise in cardiology, nutrition, pathology, pediatrics, epidemiology, and public health. T. Colin Campbell, a pioneer in the field of nutritional science and author of *The China Study* was one of the panel members.

Esselstyn challenged the group during their two-day session to determine a diet that could be given to patients that would offer optimal health, and protect against future coronary artery disease. During this session, T. Colin Campbell verbalized what many of the esteemed panel was feeling: "If we are reasonably sure of what our data from these studies are telling us, then why must we be reticent about recommending a diet which we know is safe and healthy? Scientists can no longer take the attitude that the public cannot benefit from information they are not ready for…We must tell them that a diet of roots, stems, seeds, flowers, fruit, and leaves is the healthiest diet and the only diet we can promote, endorse, and recommend." According to Esselstyn, medical organizations are equally to blame for not embracing nutritional programs backed by science. "Although they have been advising us for well over a decade that dairy products, oil, and animal fat are bad for us, and although it becomes clearer with every passing year that vascular disease, cancer, and other illness are the direct result of the toxic Western diet, these organizations just cannot bring themselves to radically change nutritional recommendations."

Americans frankly are not helping either, as many would rather continue eating their admittedly poor diet of animal fat and high fructose corn syrup, and then look for insurance companies to cover the cost of expensive drugs to combat their resulting high blood pressure, high cholesterol, and diabetes. It is often not until someone faces a serious illness that there is a willingness to change eating habits. This persistent consumer demand by Americans for their poor diet of meat, dairy, and processed carbohydrates is complex in nature. The food we eat is heavily integrated into the social fabric of our lives. Our family traditions, day-to-day activities, annual celebrations, and much more are often primarily focused around food as the central element. Food provides us with a certain familiarity and comfort. Certain foods can create bonds that are difficult to break.

A more complete discussion on why we eat the foods we do is the subject of an entire book of its own. However, one factor that likely contributes greatly to our demand for poor food is the addictive properties of certain foods. In his book *Breaking The Food Seduction*, Dr. Neal Barnard provides an excellent, in depth discussion of this topic.[6] For a more comprehensive review, I refer you to his book. For our purposes, we will cover a few salient points.

Researchers have found evidence that foods such as processed chocolate, milk, cheese and meat have been shown to stimulate similar receptors in the brain as morphine and heroin. Studies have shown that naloxone, an opiate blocking drug, can reduce cravings for processed chocolate snacks. Other studies have shown that the casein protein in milk and cheese can be further broken down to proteins called casomorphins, which have a tenth of the pain killing effect of morphine. This is why we find these foods so comforting. Individuals undergoing the intervention of our Nutritional Boot Camp have often reported typical symptoms of detoxification such as headaches, fatigue, night sweats, and irritability after removing all forms of animal flesh and dairy from their diets. It is possible that a major reason so many Americans continue to demand their poor food is because they are addicted.

> *Therefore, the best form of medicine is optimal nutrition.*

What keeps scientific evidence of nutritional excellence out of the public eye is the opinion of many that the truth would require too radical a shift from the way Americans eat today, and as such, would not be widely accepted. Rather than offer the truth about what people should be eating and offering assistance and encouragement for compliance, responsible organizations choose to take a more moderate approach. They advise people to *cut back* on meat and dairy, not eliminate it. They are advising people to use moderation. However, moderation only perpetuates the disease state.

Summary

As we discussed earlier, the body has an inherent ability to maintain itself. It can also repair and replace elements of itself. This amazing capability is made stronger with proper nutrition, which consists of plant-based foods that are minimally processed. In the context of fighting disease and maintaining health, the body has an internal system of preventing, controlling, and even reversing disease states. The food we eat must support the natural and ongoing processes the body already has in place, and maximize these operations to prevent and reverse disease. The primary way that food supports the human body is through its provision of natural biochemical substances for the body's use. Optimal food brings about optimal physical wellbeing, and with it, optimal health through disease prevention, control, or reversal. Therefore, the best form of medicine is optimal nutrition. The words of Hippocrates ring through loud and clear.

◌◍

Chapter Six
A New Approach to Health Care

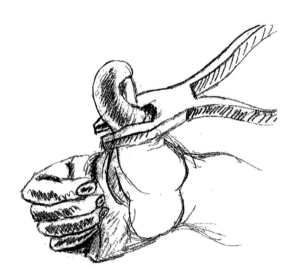

Most medical interventions involve treating patients and their symptoms to bring about relief, rather than spending time diagnosing the root cause of disease states to treat. While the example I am about to use is meant to dramatize the issue, it serves to underscore the typical approach taken in today's clinical settings. In a hypothetical scenario, a patient goes to his primary physician with a chief complaint of a swollen, tender right thumb. We will call him "Jim." He relates that he started to feel intense pain in his right thumb, immediately after a vise-grip was clamped there, two weeks ago. After a detailed medical and family history, Jim's doctor performs a complete examination of his head, eyes, ears, nose, and throat. He listens to Jim's lungs and his heart, evaluates his abdomen and extremities, and takes a close look at the right thumb, which is swollen and tender to touch.

The doctor notices the vise-grip clamped tightly in place, and examines the left thumb for comparison. After a complete assessment, he writes a prescription for Jim to take 400mg of Motrin®, three times a day. He writes another prescription for Jim to take Tylenol® with codeine, one tablet every four hours as needed for pain not relieved by the Motrin®. He discharges Jim from the office with a follow-up appointment in two weeks. Jim leaves the office with a swollen thumb, and the vise-grip still firmly in place.

He returns two weeks later, stating that while he had some initial pain relief, the pain has returned and is increasing in intensity. Jim also has new complaints. He is constipated and he has seen a decreased amount of urine he produces. His doctor orders blood tests, changes his Tylenol® with codeine to one with a larger dose of codeine, and increases his dose of Motrin®. He also prescribes a laxative to treat Jim's new symptom, constipation. Poor Jim returns two weeks later, vise-grip still in place, and he's still in pain and constipated. He now has an issue with decreased urination and shows signs of renal insufficiency (mild kidney abnormality). Jim is now referred to a kidney specialist and a gastrointestinal specialist, for his renal insufficiency and constipation, respectively. His doctor adds another narcotic medication for the pain in Jim's thumb. Nevertheless, Jim is discharged from the office with a recommended follow-up in four weeks, with the vise grip in place and the thumb even more tender and swollen.

My concern with this hypothetical scenario relates to the fact that the physician did not ever address the primary problem, which was the vise-grip on the thumb. He solely treated the symptoms of Jim's condition, which was the pain and tenderness in his thumb, the most superficial part of the problem. The pain that caused Jim to seek medical attention in the first place was only masked by the drugs prescribed, and only masked temporarily. The approach taken for his treatment resulted in the need for additional medical therapy, and required additional medical evaluation by other specialties. The problem with Jim's thumb could have been effectively treated and essentially cured by simply removing the vise-grip. This scenario may seem ridiculous, and it is, but I assure you that it is repeated on a regular basis in clinical medicine. When patients visit doctors with chronic illnesses such as hypertension, coronary heart disease, diabetes mellitus, obesity, arthritis, etc., health care professionals tend to treat only the symptoms of these diseases, while leaving the figurative vise-grip in place. The vise-grip that I am referring to in our clinical setting is the toxic and nutrient-poor standard American diet. In the vast majority of cases, medications, and therapeutic or surgical interventions are used primarily to treat the side effects of the bad food we eat.

Despite mounting evidence that the vise-grip of our chronic illnesses is our poor nutrition and lifestyle choices, we continue to apply more pills and procedures to suppress superficially the outward manifestations of these conditions. Dr. Douglas Brimner, author of *Before You Take That Pill*, estimates that approximately half of insured Americans take prescription medications, and estimates 81% of us take at least one kind of pill every day. These could be over-the-counter or prescription drugs.[1] Dr. John Abramson, author of *Overdosed American: The Broken Promise of American Medicine*, states we are pouring money into expensive drugs and medical devices that have only marginal value over more economical alternatives.[2]

While advances in medical technology have allowed for the development of less invasive medical treatments, the number of interventions in certain areas have continued to expand. Two important examples of this trend are gastric bypass surgeries and coronary artery angioplasties. A study conducted in 2005 found that over a four-year period, from 1998 to 2002, the number of gastric bypass surgeries in the U.S. climbed 450 percent.[3] In Figure 6.1 we see that in 1998, 12,775 surgeries were performed and in 2002, the annual number of these surgeries had grown to 70,256. Furthermore, the American Society for Bariatric Surgery estimates that in the following four years, the number of people electing gastric bypass surgery rose to 177,600 in 2006.[4] In 1998 approximately 539,000 angioplasties were done.[5] In 2006 the American Heart Association estimated that over 1.3 million angioplasties were performed. In both cases, the vast majority of these angioplasties were elective. Many examples are seen in other situations, such as an increasing number of younger adults and adolescents taking prescription medications regularly, resulting in an increase in the number of individuals in these age groups who will likely require more medications when they get older.

Figure 6.1

Gastric Bypass Surgeries

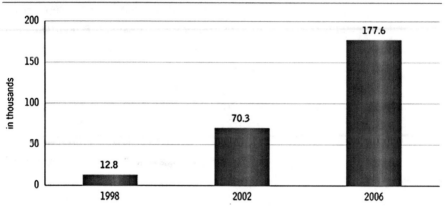

Health versus Disease

Health by definition is the general condition of the body or mind with reference to soundness and vigor. It is, in essence, freedom from disease or ailment. Disease by definition is a disorder or abnormal condition of an organ, or other part of an organism, resulting from the genetic or developmental errors, such as infection, nutritional deficiency, toxicity, or unfavorable environmental factors. Hence, health is defined by the absence of disease, which is the absence of some abnormal condition of an organ or other part of an organism.

The difficulty in defining disease in an absolute sense is related to the difficulty in determining at what point the organ or organism becomes abnormal. In clinical medicine, we have numerous diagnostic tests, clinical assessments, and physical evaluations we use to determine whether an individual has an abnormal condition. Over the centuries, the study of clinical medicine and human physiology has resulted in numerous clinical syndromes and physical assessments, developed and used to determine whether or not an individual is in a diseased state.

The point I want to make is that we are only able to define health versus disease based on limited clinical diagnostic tools. When I see someone in my office that has a normal physical exam and normal diag-nostic tests, I do not know whether this person is truly healthy or not. If I see another patient with an abnormal physical exam and diagnostic tests, I will know that the person is not healthy, but I do not know when the disease state began or the full extent it exists.

Our current clinical approach is to define disease based on an abnormal clinical finding, which often occurs long after the disease state has begun at the cellular level. For example, "Barbara" is a 50-year-old woman who sees her doctor for a routine evaluation. Over a period of days, data will be collected to assess her health using blood tests, a Pap smear, pelvic exam, breast exam, and mammogram. Barbara is a smoker and eats foods high in trans-fats. Nevertheless, all of her tests are found to be normal. Unknown to her and her doctor, she has four breast cancer cells in her left breast that were undetected in the mam-mogram. Based on Barbara's clinical evaluation she would be deemed healthy, despite the presence of cancer. The cancer would not become detectable until it is approximately one billion cells in number.

For an average growing breast cancer, it could take approximately six to eight years to become clinically detectable. During this time, Bar-bara may get consistent, normal clinical evaluations and reassurances of being healthy. She would not likely be motivated to change her lifestyle because she is cosmetically healthy, with no evident medical problems. Barbara would continue to literally feed the cancer until it becomes clinically measurable.

The above example underscores the inadequacy of our current approach, defining disease states only in terms of abnormal clinical find-ings. A paradigm shift is needed in our thinking in which we define disease states as the *pathological lifestyle* an individual has, regardless of their clinical findings. The treatment of this pathological lifestyle should be the foundation of our treatment plan, regardless of the health condi-tion the individual faces, whether it is preclinical, early stage, advanced, or even near terminal. With this approach, we will no longer overlook "removing the vise grip from the thumb."

Health Care or Sick Care

> *The treatment of this pathological lifestyle should be the foundation of our treatment plan, regardless of the health condition the individual faces, whether it is preclinical, early stage, advanced, or even near terminal.*

We are likely seeing an increase in the number of therapeutic interventions as a result of an increase in the amount of disease, which underscores an apparently single-minded or unilateral approach to treating chronic illnesses in America. In my opinion, our current system of "health care" is not one of health care at all, but one of *sick* care. It is a system primarily using pharmaceutical and therapeutic interventions for the treatment of disease. Minimal attention is given the lifestyle in general and nutrition specifically. Sick individuals are only told they must "diet and exercise" or "lose weight," if they happen to be overweight and sick. They are told their illnesses are simply "genetic," if they are sick but not overweight.

If we understand that chronic illnesses are based on an underlying biochemical or physiological imbalance that is the primary problem, then the main concern needs to be in the treatment of that primary condition, and not the superficial symptom that brings a patient into a clinical office. In my opinion, the definitive health care intervention is one that intervenes at the level of the malnourished state of most Americans.

We not only need to make a paradigm shift in our thinking, but in our actions as well. More specifically, there is need for a major paradigm shift in our current approach to the treatment of medical disease. This paradigm shift is one where we realize the need for nutritional intervention as the core, or foundation, of how we treat illness, with medical and surgical interventions used as secondary approaches. It is this nutritional intervention perspective that underscores the basic premise of this book.

For example, let's say Gina is a patient, admitted to the hospital for congestive heart failure (a condition of the heart weakening). She will be admitted to either a telemetry room where the electrical activity of her heart will be constantly monitored, or a cardiac care unit, depending on the severity of her condition. Congestive heart failure is a condition where the heart does not circulate blood adequately for the body's needs, causing fatigue and swelling. It is among the most common reasons for hospitalizations in America. Gina may also undergo expensive diagnostic procedures such as angiograms and electrical tests of the heart. She may even require the placement of a special implantable defibrillator that stimulates the lower chambers of the heart to improve their pumping function. These therapeutic interventions are excellent, and have shown to be helpful for people with this condition.

However, Gina is allowed to eat the same food she always has, with a few minimal changes. But that won't be enough to alter the factors that both started, and further perpetuates, her disease state. The only advice that individuals with a similar condition to Gina's will receive to change their current eating habits to improve their health are a few handouts encouraging them to eat a "low salt" diet. They are told about eating in "moderation" and weighing themselves. If they are smokers, they are told to stop (big revelation!). This information is given to them as basic supplemental information, as opposed to framing the foundation of the treatment plan.

Managing Health vs. Managing Sickness

So what does it mean to manage someone's health versus his or her sickness? We can best answer this by examining the current standard of care for treating an individual with type 2 diabetes. An individual—we will call him "Dave"—has elevated levels of blood sugar that are found by his physician during an examination. Likely, he will be started on oral medications in pill form to get the blood sugar down, depending on how high it is. Let's say Dave's initial fasting blood sugar is 250mg/dL.

Since his levels are above 126 mg/dL, he will be considered to have diabetes. His condition will be classified as type 2 diabetes, a condition where the body's cells do not respond normally to insulin. He likely will start taking an oral medication with the recommendation to follow a standard diabetic diet, which includes monitoring carbohydrates and fruits. He will also be told to exercise and lose weight if he is overweight.

If Dave's blood sugar remains high despite starting the oral medication, he will be given a second diabetic pill or started on insulin. The focus of his overall care will be to get his blood sugar down, well below 200mg/dL.

More and more medications will be added until the blood sugar is at or near the target range. Dave's physician will likely prescribe as many medications as necessary to "get the blood sugar down." Although reducing the blood sugar of a diabetic is a noble thing to do, this approach is inadequate because it is unilateral, and does not get to the underlying cause, which are the processed foods that Dave likely continues to eat.

With a primary nutritional approach, the first intervention for Dave would be to fully examine the foods he eats regularly to assess the extent that food is the root of the problem. In my experience, the patient's diet is the major contributing factor for type 2 diabetes, greater than 99% of the time. The management of this patient (see details in Chapter 8) would include a major change in Dave's diet, which would start by removing all forms of animal flesh, eggs, dairy, and processed foods. This initial phase of his treatment would focus on what he eats, and more importantly, what he does not eat. The psychosocial aspects of these changes would be addressed during this time. Dave would also be empowered through small group lectures, food preparation demonstrations, and informative shopping sessions. Medications would only serve as a last effort to keep Dave's health condition under control, with continued attempts to wean him off them as much as possible.

A New Role for Medications and Surgical Procedures

Looking back to Gina's situation with congestive heart failure, we would take a different approach with her as well. We would prescribe a change in her diet that would not only halt the disease state progression but would also begin reversing it. The underlying insult is removed by eliminating the unnatural food substances from Gina's diet and replacing them with natural plant-based foods. This would support her body's ability to naturally repair the damaged blood vessels, repair the damaged underlying metabolic conditions that resulted in high cholesterol, and halt the underlying conditions that would lead to future weakening of her heart. This is what brings about disease reversal and healing.

The aforementioned lifestyle intervention would be nutritionally based at first, with other components such as exercise added later. Her prescription would include the following:
- Information on specific foods to eat and those to avoid.
- Details on the best ways to prepare foods.
- Sample recipes and detailed meal plans.
- Small and large group sessions would be encouraged.
- Education on the fundamentals of optimal nutrition.
- Practical instruction on how to order at restaurants or manage food with travel schedules.

> *The vast majority of our medical care is utilized in individuals with chronic illnesses that are best treated and reversed by nutritional means.*

Similar to the example with Dave above, this intervention would enable Gina to systematically break food addictions and progressively improve her health. The educational component would further empower her with the necessary basic knowledge to maintain this lifestyle permanently.

Please do not misunderstand. I believe modern medicine has many benefits for the acutely ill individual. An example is someone who goes to his or her physician with severe chest discomfort and is found to be having a heart attack. That individual is known to benefit from acute therapeutic procedures, such as an angioplasty. My point is that such procedures should be reserved for acute illnesses. In a similar way, individuals who are affected by significant trauma from motor vehicle accidents, gunshot wounds, and the like will definitely benefit from the technological advancement of modern medicine, and the acute care of therapeutic intervention. However, the vast majority of our medical care is utilized in individuals with chronic illnesses that are best treated and reversed by nutritional means. In these settings, medications and interventions are traditionally thought to be the primary medical approach, while diet and lifestyle changes, specifically optimal nutrition, is thought to be a secondary approach. My position is that for the vast majority of these chronic illnesses, such as heart disease, diabetes mellitus, obesity, hypertension, and immune complex disorders, nutrition should be the primary source of intervention, with medications and surgical procedures being a secondary option. Our whole approach to medically treating chronic illnesses needs to shift its focus to place more emphasis in helping people control their own health states through optimal nutrition.

True Health

In our new way of thinking, true health should be a process of optimal living with continual improvement in our actions over time. We should always strive to eat better, think more positively, exercise longer and more effectively, etc. True health is more of a process than a condition or clinical test value. A person will gain true health by achieving and maintaining a lifestyle of optimal nutrition and exercise, as well as continual mental and spiritual growth. This process can occur at any age or clinical condition.

For example, an 80-year-old woman with congestive heart failure, diabetes, and high cholesterol, can achieve true health by ceasing to eat foods that are toxic to her body, and replacing them with nutritionally excellent food, exercising regularly, getting adequate sunshine, and rest. Although this person may have a weak heart on ultrasound, her truly aggressive lifestyle intervention may afford her a higher level of functioning than otherwise, with minimal or possibly no need for regular "sick care" treatments. In other words, true health for her would be to control her "disease state" with very few or no medications, few or no regular admissions to the hospital, and even very few visits to her doctor. This person would be achieving true health because her actions would be such that she is facilitating her body's ability to "heal" itself based on her new lifestyle.

On the other hand, an outwardly healthy 25-year-old woman would not have true health if she smoked, consumed the standard American diet, and was sedentary. Despite the fact that she has no detectable disease on clinical evaluation, her actions and poor lifestyle choices are contributing to her potential heart disease, cancer, kidney failure, or perhaps even lupus. This is what should define her state of disease. With this new approach to wellness, her doctor would prescribe a more aggressive lifestyle intervention during her routine well-woman evaluation that may alter her course of life.

Summary

...the major burden of chronic illnesses on our collective health could be heavily reduced or nearly eliminated by shifting our focus to our new health care model.

There is a need for revolutionary change in how we address chronic illnesses in this country and around the world. Our new paradigm will be one in which we address chronic illnesses from the perspective of our lifestyle behavior, with optimal nutrition being the central theme.

It is recognized that congenital abnormalities, physical injuries, and the like will continue to contribute to our overall health condition, and in many cases will require the best that medications and surgery have to offer. However, the major burden of chronic illnesses on our collective health could be heavily reduced or nearly eliminated, by shifting focus to our new health care model.

This model places an emphasis on first recognizing poor health as an indicator of poor lifestyle behaviors, especially poor nutritional choices. We would then aggressively intervene on that lifestyle behavior to bring about true health for people. At this point we would be providing true health care, and not just sick care.

What do we have to gain? By approaching chronic illness first with nutritional intervention, we will improve overall quality of life for people. We will improve their productivity on jobs and increase their enjoyment of day-to-day activities. We will help patients avoid costly medications and surgical procedures, allowing them to keep more money in their pockets. All it takes is the realization that true health begins in the produce section of the grocery store, not the pharmacy.

༄

Chapter Seven
The Montgomery Food
Classification System

In chapter four, we discussed the basic aspects of food, ranging from its chemical makeup to its general source of origin (plant versus animal). Our discussion in that chapter disclosed clear evidence of how foods from plant sources are superior to foods from animal sources. Furthermore, we showed evidence that the less processed foods are, the more nutritious they are. Therefore, we can move forward in our discussion with the understanding that the most nutritious foods are whole, plant-based, and that are as close to their natural state as possible. In other words, we should consume a diet of foods with three important characteristics:

- minimally processed
- whole
- plant-based

It is important to note that we do not use the labels, vegetarian, vegan, or raw vegan food to describe our food choices. This is important because, although there is considerable scientific evidence supporting the health benefits of these diets compared to diets that include meat, there are also unhealthy foods included in these diets I want to avoid. For example, deep fried, breaded okra is classified as vegan, but it may not be much healthier than sautéed chicken. To be certain that even plant-based food is healthy, we must consider how it was developed and prepared prior to our consumption. The science-based evidence that supports the position that minimally processed, whole, plant-based foods provide the most optimal nutrition is the foundation for the Montgomery Food Classification System.

Our classification system takes into consideration that foods are complex chemical structures with many features that we understand and can characterize. However, we acknowledge that foods have many more characteristics that we do not understand and hence cannot classify.

As a result, our classification system does not limit its approach to simple finite factors such as calories, sugar content, or fat content, nor arbitrary classifications such as carbohydrates, fats, or proteins. We try to assess the "global" aspects of food:

- Basic characteristics—Plant, animal, inorganic mineral (i.e. salt), or synthetic foods
- Conditions of development
- Level of processing (with the understanding that some levels of processing may be beneficial to the nutritious value of the food)
- Basic chemical characteristics
- Potential effects on the human body

The Montgomery Food Classification System (patent pending) is a proprietary system of assigning foods and other nutritional substances to categories, based on their ability to facilitate optimal human body *healing* and *function*. Various properties of foods are utilized to categorize them within the system. Five basic characteristics are described in the *Food Characteristics Design* below.

Food Characteristics Design
Food Classification Factor 1: Fundamental Characteristic of the Food
A. Plant-based—Superior
B. Natural Mineral in Inorganic State—Possibly Beneficial
C. Animal-based—Inferior
D. Synthetic—Inferior (i.e. vitamins, supplements, cloned animal products)

Food Classification Factor 2:
Type or Extent of Food Processing
Processing Category A—*Physical or Chemical Changes to the Food*

- **Group 1** *(Beneficial effects from processing)*
  a. Juicing
  b. Blending
  c. Ripening
  d. Chopping
  e. Freezing
  f. Drying (< 105°F)

- **Group 2** *(Neutral)*
  a. Poaching
  b. Warming (< 155°F)
  c. Drying/Dehydrating (< 155°F)
  d. Steaming (for duration of < 4 mins)
  e. Boiling (for duration of < 10 mins)

- **Group 3** *(Neutral)*
  a. Warming (155-200°F)
  b. Drying/Dehydrating (155-200°F)
  c. Steaming (for duration of 4-10 mins)
  d. Boiling (for duration of 10-45 mins)

- **Group 4** *(Neutral to mildly adverse effects from processing)*
  a. Warming (temp > 200°F)
  b. Drying/Dehydrating (temp > 200°F)
  c. Steaming (for duration of > 10 mins)
  d. Boiling (for duration of > 45 mins)

- **Group 5** *(Adverse effects from processing)*
  a. Jarring
  b. Canning
  c. Baking (temp > 400°F)

- **Group 6** *(Very adverse effects from processing)*
  a. Sautéing (or stir frying)
  b. Frying (deep, or shallow in a pan)
  c. Grilling

     d. Microwaving

     e. Use of heat or chemical solvents to extract or separate compo-
nents of a whole food (example; extracted vegetable oils)

Processing Category B—*The Extent of Mixing or Combining of the Food (No direct application of Category B will be used in this version of the classification system)*

- Mono-Food—One ingredient
- Pauci-Food—Five ingredients or less
- Complex Food Greater than five ingredients

**Food Classification Factor 3:
Baseline Nutritional and/or Chemical Characteristics of the Food**

1. **Glycemic Index**—a major sub-factor
   A. Low < 55
   B. Medium 56 to 70
   C. High > 70

2. **Nutrient Density**—a major sub-factor
   A. High Nutrient Density (Aggregate Nutrient Density Index > 90)ı
   B. Medium to Low Nutrient Density (Aggregate Nutrient Density Index < 90)

3. **Nutrient Content**—phytonutrient, vitamin, and mineral—minor sub-factor; a subcomponent of Nutrient Density

4. **Glycemic Load**—minor sub-factor; a subcomponent of Glycemic Index

5. **Macromolecular Profile**—percentage fats, carbohydrates, and proteins—a minor subfactor

Food Classification Factor 4:
Origin of Food's Development
A. Development in "Wild Conditions" remote from polluted environments—Superior
B. Naturally Cultivated (remote from polluted environments)—Good
C. Unnaturally Cultivated—Inferior.

The above classification scheme is not meant to be memorized in detail. The purpose for providing it here is to show the various factors that are used to classify foods into the various food levels. Notice the absence of factors such as caloric content, portion size, protein amount, etc.

The Food Classification System
A food classification system on a scale of 0 to 10 was devised for the purpose of placing foods in groups ranging from the healthiest (level 0) to the most "toxic" (level 10). This 0 to 10 scale was devised to eliminate the need for reading food labels, counting calories or points, or measuring portion sizes. Certain food levels of similar health value are grouped into zones (detoxification zone, maintenance zone, and disease progression zone) for further simplification.

Under each food level below is a general description of the type of foods in that group and details on how the food is developed or prepared. Below the description in each level is a list of examples of foods that meet the criteria for that level. Similar to the Food Characteristics Design, this section is intended for use as a reference source, rather than a long list of items to be memorized.

Figure 7.1

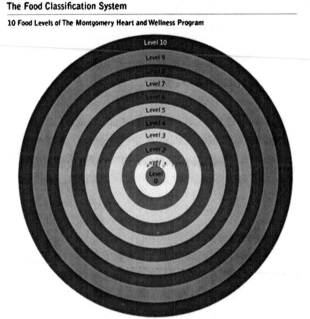

The Food Classification System

10 Food Levels of The Montgomery Heart and Wellness Program

The Food Levels in Detail
Food Level 0

Food Level 0 may be the primary starting point or the core of all of the food levels. This level may consist of raw or "live" foods in a liquid form. As such, Food Level 0 may theoretically contain live enzymes, proteins, minerals, and other nutrients that are easily absorbed by the body, with minimal energy expenditure. As an example, water may be considered to be a Food Level 0 food, even though it does not contain substances that are classically thought of as nutrients. This is because it is a super nutrient itself. Other foods in Food Level 0 may include naturally fermented beverages from fruits and vegetables, freshly blended fruits and vegetables (e.g., in the form of fruit and vegetable smoothies), freeze-dried or dehydrated foods at a temperature that is less than 100°F, and reconstituted in water. In theory, Food Level 0 food consumption would allow for the body to get nourishment in an energy conservative manner. Foods eaten in this way allow nutrients to be easily absorbed by the body. For example, the body can more easily absorb nutrients from liquids, than solids. Therefore, liquids may allow for maximal cleansing and rebuilding of body cells and tissues.

NOTE: Juices in Food Level 0 are juiced fresh without pasteurization. The juices in Level 0 are not pasteurized.

Examples of foods in Food Level 0 include:
Miscellaneous Beverages:
Water
Raw Lemonade (15 oz. of unpasteurized lemon juice/ 1 to 1 ½ cups Agave Nectar/ dilute to one gallon)
Apple Cider Vinegar
Kombucha
Liquid Blue-Green Algae
Organic Green Tea
Organic Black Tea
Organic, non-boiled, herbal tea

Basic Vegetable Juices: 16 oz. per serving:
Carrot, beet (include beet tops)
Carrot & celery with tops
Carrot, apple, & celery
Carrot, cucumber, parsley, spinach
Carrot, celery, broccoli, garlic (1 clove or more to suit)
Carrot, celery, spinach, beet, cabbage, red pepper
Carrot, red pepper, 1-chili pepper
Carrot, beet, parsley, ginger, garlic, 1-3 pieces of chili pepper

Combination Juices:
Carrot & apple
Carrot, apple, ginger
Carrot, apple, broccoli
Apple, beet
Sweet potato, beet, apple
Fennel bulb, apple, ginger, mint
Pineapple, celery, apple
Cucumber, celery, apple, mint, parsley
Grapefruit, lemon, olive oil, cayenne, garlic
Pineapple, cucumber, apple
Carrot, beet, garlic, wheatgrass

Fruit Juices:
Orange & grapefruit
Orange & strawberry
Orange, lime, strawberry
Apple, ginger, wheatgrass
Orange, pineapple, strawberry
Apple, strawberry, ginger

Subcategories of Food Level 0

Subcategory I: *Glycemic Index*
A. Glycemic Index of d" 55
B. Glycemic Index between 56 and 70
C. Glycemic Index greater than 70

Subcategory II: *Nutrient Density*
A. High Nutrient Density (ANDI of d" 90)
B. Low Nutrient Density (ANDI of > 90)

Subcategory III: *Origin of Development or Growth*

A. Harvested from a "Wild" Environment
B. Cultivated or Grown in an "Organic" Environment (free of pollution, synthetic substances)
C. Cultivated or Grown in an environment of pollution and/or synthetic chemical substances. For example, a food, such as blue-green algae, Aphanizomenon flos-aqua (E3-live®) in its liquid form, has a glycemic index (GI) of less than 50, which means that it is a Subcategory I-A food. The blue-green algae also has a high nutrient density, which means that it is also a Subcategory II-A food. If the blue-green algae is harvested from its wild, natural environment, it is also a Subcategory III-A food. Using these subcategories, the food level categorizer will classify blue-green algae as a Level 0 AAA food. Organic raw pineapple juice (with a glycemic index greater than 70, and a medium nutrient density) would be a Level 0 CBB.

Food Level 1

Food Level 1 may consist of raw foods in a solid state that have a high nutrient density and low glycemic index. Vegetables in this group may have dark, rich colors and are very low in fat and starch. Sprouts, brightly colored berries, grapes, and cruciferous vegetables (which may not have dark rich colors) are also be part of Food Level 1, because of their high nutritional density. Foods in this level are prepared and eaten in their "raw" state.

Examples of Foods in Level 1 include:

Acai Berries
Alfalfa Sprouts
Algae
Arugula
Bean Sprouts
Blackberries
Blueberries
Bok Choy
Broccoli
Broccolini (Asparition)
Broccoli Sprouts
Brussels sprouts
Cabbage (red or green)
Cauliflower
Celery
Chinese cabbage
Chives
Collard greens
Daikon
Dandelion
Garlic
Goji Berries
Herbs (dried or fresh)
Kale
Kohlrabi
Leeks

Mushrooms (raw)
Mustard greens
Onions
Peppers—all types (bell peppers, jalapeño
peppers, paprika, cayenne peppers, etc.)
Plums
Pomegranate Seeds
Radishes
Raspberries
Rutabaga
Sea Vegetation (Sea Weed)
Shallot
Strawberries
Turnips
Watercress
Welsh onion (Green onion)

Food Level 2

In Level 2, fruits and vegetables are added that have a medium to low glycemic index or a medium to low nutrient density. Level 2 foods are prepared and eaten in their "raw" state.

Examples of Foods in Level 2 include:

Asparagus
Beets
Carrots
Cucumbers
Eggplant
Green Beans
Tomatoes
Squash—Summer (crookneck, zucchini, etc.)
Squash—Winter (pumpkin, butternut
squash, acorn squash, etc.)
Sweet Potatoes (or yams)

Food Level 3

Food Level 3 may consist of "raw" nongrain, plant-based foods that have a high glycemic index.

Examples of foods in Food Level 3 include:
Apples
Apricot
Bananas
Cantaloupe
Corn, raw, organic
Dates
Grapefruit
Grapes
Honeydew Melon
Idaho Potatoes (raw, organic)
Kiwi
Mangos
Nectarine
Oranges
Peach
Pear
Pineapples
Prunes
Raisins
Red Potatoes
Watermelon

A low glycemic index may include foods with a glycemic index lower than 55. A high nutrient density food may include those that have an aggregate nutrient density index that is greater than 90. If the foods have a low glycemic index and a high nutrient density, they are categorized into Food Level 1. A low to mid-glycemic index food may include foods that have a glycemic index between 0-70. The low to mid-nutrient density foods may include those that have an aggregate nutrient density index that is less than 90. If the foods have these characteristics, they are categorized in Food Level 2. High glycemic index foods include those that have a glycemic index greater than 70. If foods have these characteristics, they are categorized into Food Level 3.

Food Level 4
Foods that are dried, dehydrated, or warmed at a temperature less than 155°F, or steamed or boiled for a short duration are categorized as

Food Level 4. A short duration for steaming foods includes a time that is less than 4 minutes, and a short duration for boiling foods includes a time that is less than 10 minutes. Level 4 foods include lightly steamed, soaked, sprouted, dehydrated, or warmed fruits, vegetables, legumes or beans, and grains. Light processing includes 4 minutes or less for steaming, and 10 minutes or less for boiling. Raw avocados and other raw plant-based foods that have a high fat content (with the exception of nuts) are included in Level 4. Inorganic unprocessed minerals are added to this food level also, for example, sea salt.

Examples of Foods in Level 4 include:
Steamed or blanched (4 minutes or less) vegetables listed in Food Levels 1-3
Avocados (raw)
Beans—dried or frozen (kidney, red, lima, navy, garbanzo, soy)
Black-eyed Peas
Edamame (soybeans)
Gluten Free Pasta
Olives
Sea Salt—Celtic
Sea Salt—Himalayan (can also be part of a Food Level 1 vegetable soup)
Split Pea Soup (sprouted and cooked for a short duration)

Food Level 5
Foods that are warmed, dried, or dehydrated at temperatures between 155°F and 200°F, and steamed or boiled for a medium duration are categorized as level 5. A medium duration for steaming foods consists of a time duration between 4 and 10 minutes, and a medium duration for boiling foods consists of a time duration between 10 and 45 minutes. Typical foods in level 5 include greens, beans and legumes, starches, including grains, bean or mixed vegetable soups, and other fruit and vegetables that are boiled for up to 45 minutes, or oven warmed (temperature between 155°F and 200°F). Cooked fats and extracted oils or nuts are excluded. Food Level 5 may not include high fat foods (i.e., foods with fat content of greater than 20% per unit caloric content) that are cooked at any time.

Examples of Foods in Level 5 include:
Ezekiel Bread
Oats (steel cut oats, minimally processed)—cooked
Quinoa (soaked, lightly blanched, or steamed)
Pasta, gluten-free
Rice, brown (not white rice)
Rice, wild—cooked
Rice Crackers
Sprouted Grain Bread (Ezekiel, Manna brand)
Sweet Potato—warmed (not white potatoes)

Food Level 6

Food Level 6 is the same as Food Level 5, except for the increased time of steaming and boiling. Foods that are baked, warmed, dried, or dehydrated at a temperature greater than 200°F, or steamed or boiled for a long duration, and have up to 20% fat per unit serving are categorized in Food Level 6. A long duration for steaming foods includes a time greater than 10 minutes, and a long duration for boiling foods includes a time greater than 45 minutes. Food Level 6 may also include raw, organic nuts and seeds.

Examples of Foods in Level 6:
Blue Corn Chips (baked)—organic, less than 20% fat by caloric content
Brazil nuts—raw and organic
Gluten Free Crackers
Gluten Free Pancakes
Gluten Free Waffles
Hemp Seeds—raw and organic
Oatmeal (standard processed)
Pecans—raw and organic
Pumpkin Seeds (Pepitas)—raw and organic
Rice Crackers
Sunflower Seeds—raw and organic
Tahini—raw and organic
Tamari

Tempeh
Tofu
Vegetable Pasta
Veggie Burgers
Walnuts—raw and organic

Food Level 7

Food Level 7 may add clean fish to Food Levels 0 through 6. Clean fish may include all types of fish, except fish classified as shellfish, catfish, or fish that are likely to have significant levels of mercury or other contaminants. The fish in Food Level 7 needs to be wild caught, and may not be farm-raised. Fish in Food Level 7 may be raw (e.g., sushi or sashimi), lightly steamed, or poached for a duration of 8 minutes or less. Food Level 7 may also include plant-based foods that have been moderately processed or have natural additives. Processed or heated vegetable oils or cooked foods with more than 20% fat by calorie may also be included in Food Level 7. Synthetic foods considered to be nutraceutical agents with the addition of natural additives may also be included in Food Level 7.

Examples of Foods in Level 7 include:
Almond Milk—boxed, pasteurized
Canned Beans
Canned Tomato Sauce
Coconut Milk Canned
Egg Whites
Flounder
Sardines
Salmon
Sole
Trout
Tilapia

Food Level 8

Food Level 8 is the same as Food Level 7, except it includes wild game meats, clean fish processed to a greater extent than described in Level 7 (lightly steamed or poached for a duration of greater than 8 minutes), and plant based foods that are grilled or heavily processed.

Food Level 8 may also include carbohydrates with white flour, white rice, or natural foods that have been stripped of their natural components. Synthetic foods in Food Level 8 include pharmaceutical agents.

Examples of Foods in Level 8 include:
Deer
Buffalo
Soft Drinks
Sports Drinks
Waffles (processed, white flour)
White Bread
White Flour Pastas
White Flour Tortillas

Food Level 9
   Animal-based foods that include domestically raised animals, excluding beef and pork, and plant-based foods that are sautéed, stir-fried, medium or deep fried, or microwaved are categorized in Food Level 9. Other animal based foods include all other types of fish (i.e., "uncleaned" fish), such as shellfish, catfish, or a fish that is likely to have significant levels of mercury or other contaminants. Food Level 9 may also include foods containing dairy products (foods containing animal milk or derivatives thereof).

Examples of Foods in Level 9 include:
Cheese—all types, organic, free range
Chicken—all types, organic, free range
Cow's Milk—all types, organic, free range
Goat's Milk—all types, organic, free range
Goat
Imitation Cheese
Lamb
Turkey
Yogurt

   Food Level 10 may include all other types of animal-based foods, and plant-based foods prepared in any way. Accordingly, Food Level 10 may include all other types of processed foods of any kind, with any

type of chemical preservative. Synthetic foods that may be considered
pharmaceutical agents are listed below.

Cheese—all types, non-organic
Clams
Cow's Milk—non-organic
Crab
Fried foods of any kind
Iodized Salt
Lobster
Meat (non-organic)—Poultry, Lamb,
Goat
Meat (organic or non-organic)—Beef and Pork
Oysters
Pork
Shark
Shrimp
Soda—diet or regular
Steak
Sugared cereals
Swordfish
Tuna
Whole Eggs—cooked or raw

Prescription Medications in General—blood pressure medications,
cholesterol medications, etc.*

Over-the-counter medications—pain relievers, decongestants, etc.*

* Note: *While prescription medications are listed above as being in Level 10,
it is understood that certain medications cannot be discontinued without a
physician's supervision. Certain medications should not be abruptly discontinued. Hence, for the purposes of nutritional detoxification, only non-prescription
pharmacological substances should be discontinued when possible. Prescription substances should be considered to be anything recommended by a
treating licensed physician, whether or not it requires a written prescription.*

It should be reiterated that this overall nutritional design should not be memorized, but rather used as a reference for understanding how foods should be classified from a health perspective. This approach to classifying food does not intend to remove the spontaneity and social pleasure from eating. To the contrary, many of our wellness clients find the application of this system to be more liberating, as it does not require calorie counting or portion measuring.

In the next chapter, we will discuss and show how this system is prescribed in the food prescription approach to health maintenance.

൭

Chapter Eight
Food Prescriptions for Illness Recovery and Wellness

Patients I see in my office often tell me about encounters they have had with other physicians, who have instructed them to improve their health by losing weight through diet and exercise. These patients are often frustrated because the usual discussion around the need to diet and exercise comes in the form of broad recommendations, without specific instructions of what to do and how to do it. This lack of precision in a sense abandons patients in the middle of a battlefield of media inputs for how to make lifestyle changes. We may assume as medical professionals that the proper way to diet and exercise is common knowledge. Or we may falsely believe that any change our patient makes is better than nothing. Experience in my own practice proves otherwise. Patients left to determine their own approach often wind up pursuing fad diets, gym memberships, expensive trainers, or even loosely structured walking clubs, all advertising quick results. Sadly, many of these well-meaning efforts turn out to be futile, with no significant benefits.

This becomes very discouraging, leading many to return quickly to their destructive eating habits because it is what they know. As health care professionals, we need to recognize that a broad, nonspecific recommendation for someone to simply diet and exercise is at best meaningless, and at its worst, insulting. Such advice without further instruction would be akin to recommending someone take "pills" for their hypertension, diabetes, and high cholesterol, without any description of medication names or dosages. Moreover, it would be considered malpractice for a physician to make such broad, nonspecific recommendations in regards to prescription medications or procedures, without precise instructions on how to comply. Why would we consider a recommendation to generically diet and exercise be any different? We care for individuals in our clinic with conditions ranging from "normal health" to end stage heart failure or advanced lung disease. In my experience, I have found it important to tailor nutritional recommendations to the specific needs of the individual based on their health condition, social environment, etc. A simple recommendation of eating fresh plant based foods is not adequate for individuals with advanced disease. Over the years, I have developed an approach to using nutrition in a therapeutic way. The Montgomery Food Classification System describes nutritional value in a more global manner. The experience I gathered over many years of using this classification system for nutritional intervention has allowed me to treat successfully the health conditions of hundreds of my patients and clients. Their positive outcomes have been a direct result of specific recommendations that form the foundation of *The Food Prescription for Better Health*.

My goal is to teach others how to implement new, healthier eating habits. My approach fills the void left by others, who are still offering only broad instructions for patients to diet and exercise. *The Food Prescription* provides the structure people desperately need to combat chronic illness and disease effectively.

Baseline Health Conditions to Consider

In clinical medicine, we vary our approach to patient treatment according to age, health status, and our assessment of a patient's level of clinical stability. For example, an individual who comes into my office for a simple health screening will be evaluated and treated in a much different way than someone who comes into the office sweaty, short of breath, and collapses. In the same way, our clinical intervention and medical therapeutics vary according to the severity and acuity of a person's health condition. So should our nutritional intervention and therapeutics.

The specific nutritional interventions I recommend for treating various health conditions depend on the person's baseline health status. There are five general health condition categories to be considered. It should be noted that the categories described below are based on standard clinical assessments, utilizing state-of-the-art medical technologies at the time of this writing. Additionally, the new approach of considering adverse lifestyle behavior as part of the disease state is also applied here.

Category One—An individual in this category has optimal health, wellness, and fitness for their age. An example is a high school-aged competitive athlete, without any known medical problems, and in an excellent level of fitness. This person has no notable adverse lifestyle habits other than consuming the standard American diet. Another example is an adult nonathlete, without any known medical problems, with a normal physical examination, but perhaps who may have poor eating habits (regular consumption of fried foods, soft drinks, and candies).

Category Two—An individual with suboptimal health, but no requirements for medical or surgical therapies would exemplify this category. This individual could be a weekend jogger with borderline elevated blood pressure but no other medical problems. Another example is the mother of an infant with a prior history of mildly elevated blood sugar during her pregnancy.

Category Three—An individual in this group would have a chronic stable or slowly declining health condition that requires medical or surgical therapies. An example is a 45-year-old woman with diabetes mellitus and high blood pressure, requiring an increase in her medications. Another example is a 50-year-old man with high cholesterol and increasing fatigue over the past year.

Category Four—This individual would have chronic, moderately declining health conditions, requiring an increase in existing medical and surgical therapies. For example, a 65-year-old retired executive with recurrent chest discomfort six years after undergoing a four-vessel coronary artery bypass surgery, and currently requiring the placement of two coronary stents in his heart to treat new chest pain symptoms. Another example is a 55-year-old woman with a known condition of congestive heart failure, who, after seeing her cardiologist for worsening shortness of breath, is recommended for admission to the hospital for intravenous heart medications and an implantable defibrillator.

Category Five—This individual would have an acutely decompensated medical illness, with a rapidly declining health status, requiring urgent or emergent medical or surgical intervention. An example is a 45-year-old man with diabetes, high blood pressure, and severely elevated cholesterol, who is being rushed to the emergency department for sudden onset of severe chest discomfort, sweatiness, and shortness of breath. Another example is a 49-year-old woman with known hypertension, diabetes, and heart failure, who is being rushed to the emergency department and being placed on an artificial ventilator for acute shortness of breath due to the buildup of fluid in her lungs.

It should be emphasized that the different categories represent different *levels* of illness, not different diagnoses. Although certain disease types were used for examples, any disease can be substituted in the various categories. Hence, it is the clinical severity of a person's illness that determines which category they are placed, rather than their specific diagnosis.

Food Prescriptions

The foundation of creating food prescriptions will lie in our Food Classification Design, combined with our baseline health assessment categories as described above. The individual in **Category 1** with optimal health and wellness will be recommended to follow food levels 0 to 6.

Ideally, an individual in this category will consume food in this classification range indefinitely with annual detoxification periods for 3 to 4 weeks. An individual in **Category 2** would start with a detoxification period of at least 4 weeks. Subsequent to this time, they will progress to a maintenance phase for approximately 3 months. They should then evaluate their condition and decide whether they should repeat a detoxification period or remain in maintenance longer. The decision to remain in maintenance or return to detoxification should be based on whether or not their health improvements achieved during detoxification have been maintained.

Alternatively, the individual could carefully evaluate what they are eating in levels 5 and 6 to make sure that overly processed plant-based foods are not being added inadvertently. A common mistake I see individuals make is to focus on not consuming any animal products, but forget to exclude plant-based foods with cooked oils.

As we progress in severity of baseline health conditions, our food prescriptions will need to be more aggressive to control and reverse adverse health states. Therefore, individuals with chronically stable, slowly declining health conditions that require medical therapies and surgeries, **Category 3**, will be recommended to initiate a detoxification phase from 0 to 3 for at least four weeks. These individuals should have their regular physician monitoring any medications they are taking while going through detox. From my experience, most people will need to reduce dosages or even eliminate certain medical therapies as a result of the detox process. Cholesterol and diabetes medications are good examples of drugs my patients have been able to reduce or eliminate, as their health begins to improve with nutritional intervention.

In many cases, it may be advisable for individuals in this category to remain in this range for longer (possibly two to six months). After that time, it will be recommended they transition into levels 0 to 6, and then stay in that range indefinitely. Furthermore, they will be recommended to return to a detoxification phase within a few months if their initial health improvements are lost.

Someone in **Category 4** who has a chronic, moderately declining health condition, requiring increased medical or surgical therapies would be recommended to undergo a detoxification phase of 0 to 3 for 4 weeks, but then could relax into a maintenance phase of levels 0 to 4 for a prolonged period of time. Someone in this category should strongly consider an eating lifestyle of 0 to 4 as their maintenance phase. Finally, someone in **Category 5** would be initially placed on food level 0 until their illness stabilizes, and then will receive a recommendation to remain at levels 0 to 3 for an additional 6 months. Subsequent to this time, they would be recommended to go to levels 0 to 4 for their maintenance.

Modification of each regimen will be made based on an individual's tolerance and clinical response within each health category.

Applying this therapeutic approach has been successful in reversing deteriorating trends for hundreds of patients and clients I have treated. The high rate of success has been due to the ability of the body to heal itself in the context of optimal nutrition. Additionally, the step-by-step instructions we give people allows for easy compliance. We have found repeatedly that patients achieve almost immediate success and improvement in their health conditions and have validated this approach as an easy method to follow. I routinely hear comments from patients that they are happy not to have to count calories, carbs, or points, perhaps for the first time in their lives!

Figure 8.1

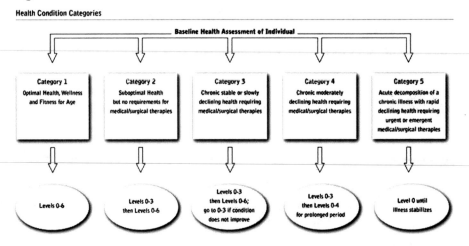

Health Condition Categories

Figure 8.2

Zones	Detoxification Zone	Slow Healing or Maintenance Zone	Disease Development or Progression Zone
Food Levels	Food Level 0	Food Level 4	Food Level 7
	Food Level 1	Food Level 5	Food Level 8
	Food Level 2	Food Level 6	Food Level 9
	Food Level 3		Food Level 10

How to Get Started

> *No part of this book is meant to replace the medical advice and care of your physician. You should always consult your physician prior to starting any lifestyle modification program.*

Patients and clients are generally introduced to the program through a Nutritional Boot Camp that is conducted within my health and wellness program over a period of four weeks. I am now broadening my reach to help those who live far away from my facility to achieve the same excellent results. *Boot Camp* is formally defined as a camp for training U.S. Navy or Marine recruits. The phrase is also frequently used to define exercise programs for physical conditioning. These training programs are generally intense, time limited programs designed to "jump start" an individual's physical conditioning level. My *Nutritional Boot Camp* is a similarly intense, time limited program, but utilizes a *nutritional regimen* rather than an exercise regimen.

Nutritional Boot Camp can be characterized in the following way:
- An intense nutritional regimen
- Has a finite period of time (usually four weeks but could be shorter or longer)
- Contributes to physical conditioning through accelerated detoxification
- Does not require exercise (individuals can continue their routine exercise regimes or rest if needed)
- Facilitates overall improved health by allowing for disease prevention and reversal
- Provides group support for choosing more healthy food and lifestyle choices, by sharing experiences, monitoring progress, and receiving feedback.

The program is a finite period of time in which an individual removes all "toxic" foods from his or her diet and consumes only "nutritionally excellent" foods, specifically, foods within levels 0 to 3. The resulting physical conditioning that occurs is **accelerated detoxification**. Detoxification is simply the process in which the body clears unnatural substances (toxins) from within.

Health Benefits of Detoxification
The body has the ability to detoxify itself regularly, unless it is bombarded by toxins found in the standard American diet. When this happens, harmful substances accumulate in the body over time and result in accelerated aging, chronic illnesses, and fatigue. These conditions are further exacerbated if organs critical for detoxification (the liver, the

kidneys, the heart) are damaged as a result of these excess toxins. It is generally recommended that anyone who wants to control, improve, or reverse a particular chronic illness should help their bodies more effectively remove excess toxins from within its cells and tissue layers by starting a detoxification program. My patients often approach me with various substances they have bought "off the shelf " that were recommended as good agents for detoxification. My usual response is to remind them that detoxification is something the body does, and not a product one consumes.

The first step in detoxification is to remove toxic substances from the foods you consume and allow the body to detoxify itself. Simply stated, the first step in detox is to *not tox*. As mentioned earlier, foods in levels 0 through 3 are categorized in the detoxification zones. Foods in these levels are substances that are plant-based and very close to their natural state of development.

It is important that you stay within the detoxification range for a period of about three to four weeks to allow your body to recover fully. 100% compliance with this approach is very important. Remind yourself that it is *only* four weeks. (For more information on food classifications, see Chapter Seven.) When you nourish your body within this zone, I know from clinical experience that people undergo significant changes in their body composition, which includes not only weight loss, but removal of excess fluid, reduction of inches from their waistline and neck, as well as improvement in blood pressure, skin tone, and various other physical conditions.

It's important to note that people who are thin, with a normal BMI do not lose a significant amount of weight. For people committed to following our detoxification program, we have also seen great improvements in reductions to overall inflammation. This is measured by significant decreases we see in C-reactive protein (CRP), a factor found in blood samples, which tells us the relative amount of inflammation present. In a similar way, people see a significant reduction in their cholesterol levels, as well as a reduction in their blood pressure. For more information, see our *Nutritional Boot Camp Results* section in Chapter 9.

I find it very rewarding to watch people go through an amazing transformation during the detoxification phase, starting from a point of being focused on what they will have to give up, to a place at the end of four weeks where they show a sense of peace about them as a result of finding improved health. People tell us frequently with a lot of excitement of improved energy levels, increases in their ability to exercise, as well as improvements to their mood and overall psyche. After four weeks of eating foods in Levels 0 to 3, many also tell us about significant reductions in their food cravings for dairy, meat, and processed carbohydrates. All of these improvements are truly life changing.

What to Expect During Detoxification

Detoxification symptoms—both physical and mental—may appear when you alter your lifestyle by starting something new, such as changing your diet or exercising, or by discontinuing a current habit, such as eating chocolate or drinking coffee. These symptoms include headache, stomachache, cough, diarrhea, skin eruptions (rash), clogged sinus, and fever, as well as feeling rundown and irritable. The symptoms may be of short duration and slight irritation, or they could last longer and cause you considerable discomfort.

The symptoms people experience during detoxification may seem contradictory to what you think might happen when you start a healthy eating program. However, when considering this contradiction carefully, it is easy to understand. When you detox, you begin to remove toxins from the body's cells and tissues, and transfer them through the bloodstream to be eliminated from the body. Your body reacts to the circulating toxins with an allergic-like response. Eliminating foods with addictive properties from your diet, like caffeine and dairy may result in withdrawal symptoms, like loss of energy, headache, or sore muscles.

Symptoms are generally more pronounced during the first week, and then subside as your body becomes used to your new pattern of eating. Think about how you might have experienced this after playing a sport you're not used to. Afterwards, you might feel tired and have sore muscles, but then feel better over the next day or two. The same is true for people eliminating toxins from their bodies.

Possible Side Effects during Detoxification
- Clogged sinuses
- Constipation
- Cough
- Diarrhea
- Fatigue
- Fever
- Flu symptoms
- Cold symptoms
- Gas
- Headache
- Irritability
- Moodiness
- Skin rash
- Stomachache

General Approach to Prepare for Detoxification
- Notify your physician of your plans to start the detoxification program.
- Review all of your medications with your physician and discuss the possible need to make medication changes during the program (i.e. the need to decrease or discontinue diabetes or high blood pressure medications).
- Continue to monitor your health conditions as you have done prior to starting the program (i.e. blood sugar checks or blood pressure checks).
- Discuss the potential detoxification reactions with your physician.
- Review the food level system carefully and start at a higher food level (a less aggressive detoxification) if you consume a poor diet or consume substances such as alcohol, tobacco, etc.

Foods to Avoid During Detoxification
(Memorize This List)
- All forms of animal flesh (pork, beef, chicken, turkey, fish, etc.)
- Dairy products (any animal's milk or derivatives thereof including yogurt, cream, cheese, butter, ice cream, sherbet, etc.)
- Eggs and egg products

- Processed cereals (oatmeal, corn flakes, grits, etc.)
- Cooked grains (rice, pasta, bread, corn, wheat, or foods with wheat gluten such as breads)
- Soft drinks, pasteurized fruit juices, alcohol, coffee, etc.
- Any other pasteurized beverages
- Any foods that are fried, baked, steamed, grilled, boiled, micro-waved, roasted, or sautéed

Maintenance Phase

After a four-week detoxification period, we recommend for people without severe major medical problems, and who have achieved significant improvement in their current medical condition to proceed to the maintenance phase. During maintenance, we recommend that people eat the vast majority of their foods within Levels 0 to 4, with the occasional addition of foods in Levels 5 and 6. This will allow you to eat a wider variety of foods, while continuing to get the best nutrition possible.

We advise everyone to detox at least once every 12 months. Depending on your health condition, the frequency of detoxification may need to occur more frequently, particularly if you have significant problems that require a more aggressive approach. If you have severe health problems, you may have to remain at Levels 0 to 3 indefinitely. I know a number of healthy individuals who elect to eat at Levels 0 to 4 only because it allows them to feel their most energetic. Individuals who are in relatively good physical health and only want to maintain their health condition, or slightly improve their physical fitness level, will need to go through detoxification less frequently.

Final Points

The weekly meal plan in Figure 8.3 and supporting sample recipes found in Appendix B are meant to serve as guides to use during the detoxification period. Some of the recipes are a bit complex, but are primarily intended to serve as examples of the amount of variety that can be achieved. Eating simply five apples, three peaches, and two bananas for breakfast, followed by a large bowl of raw spinach with diced tomatoes, alfalfa sprouts, and avocado slices, with a large fruit and vegetable smoothie (for example the Spinach Power Smoothie) for dinner would be an excellent and easy detoxification meal plan. Feel free to make changes to your liking.

It is very important that you memorize the Foods to Avoid List. You need to avoid those foods, 100% of the time—99.999999999% is not enough! In our Nutritional Boot Camp classes we have a motto— "Not a bite, not a crumb, not a drop." Participants hear, over and over again that, NOTHING in the Foods to Avoid List should be consumed.

Remember the detoxification symptoms I highlighted earlier might occur for you. If so, treat them with rest and hydration. Consult your physician if your symptoms seem to go on too long or are severe. Lastly, enjoy the journey!

Figure 8.3

Sample Weekly Food Plan (see Appendix C for detailed recipes)

Meal	Sunday	Monday	Tuesday	Wednesday	Thursday	Friday	Saturday
Morning	Early Morning Hydration	Early Morning Hydration	Early Morning Hydration	Early Morning Hydration	Early Morning Hydration	Early Morning Hydration	Early Morning Hydration
	E3 Live Shot*	E3 Live Shot*	E3 Live Shot*	E3 Live Shot*	E3 Live Shot*	E3 Live Shot*	E3 Live Shot*
Mid-Morning	Green Power Smoothie	Raisins & Sprouts	Fruit Salad w/ Fruit Dressing	Green Power Smoothie	Spinach Power Smoothie	Super Green Meal	Spinach Power Smoothie
Lunch	Broccoli, Cauliflower, & Raisin Salad	Fresh Spring Mix Garden Salad	Green Power Smoothie	Fresh Spring Mix Garden Salad	Broccoli, Cauliflower, & Raisin Salad	Green Power Smoothie	Fresh Spring Mix Garden Salad
Afternoon	Fresh Organic Bananas	Organic Raisins	Raisins & Sprouts	Green Fruit Salad	Fresh Organic Bananas	Raisins & Sprouts	Organic Raisins
Evening	Kale Salad	Carrot Tuna	Seaweed Salad	Sweet Potato Salad	Hijiki & Sprouts	Kale Salad	Carrot Tuna

E3Live® is blue green algae grown in Klamath Lake, Oregon. We use it regularly with our wellness clients and clinical patients with great results.

Chapter Nine
Saving Lives with Nutritional Intervention

The Montgomery Heart and Wellness Clinic uses various interactive programs to help people improve their health through natural means. The *Nutritional Boot Camp* is one such program that has been applied with great success. The *Boot Camp* is a miniature curriculum, consisting of five, three-hour weekly sessions. Individuals sign up in groups that meet at our facility.

Each session consists of a PowerPoint presentation that covers one of several topics, such as the details of the food classification system, the physiology of the body, food toxins, and detailed instructions on how to make healthy choices when ordering at a restaurant. Each session includes a food preparation demonstration, as well as a final session that includes an instructional supermarket shopping tour. Participants follow the nutritional detoxification program outlined in Chapter Seven of this book for the entire four weeks. Our Nutritional Boot Camp participants come to us with a variety of health conditions, ranging from those without any clinically identified health problems to those with severe conditions, classified as end-stage, or near endstage. A basic health and wellness assessment is provided as part of the Boot Camp. This allows the participants to track their results and to experience for themselves the effectiveness of the program. We perform many of the standard tests people have done routinely during a medical evaluation. The categories of tests we perform include:

- Weight and BMI (Body Mass Index)
- Blood Pressure and Heart Rate
- Inflammation
- Cholesterol
- Blood Sugar
- Kidney Function

By looking at these categories one at a time, I can provide more insight into what these tests tell us as medical professionals about someone's overall starting and ending health conditions. I will also share the results of our Nutritional Boot Camp sessions, which represents the actual results experienced by over 200 individuals. An exception is for results shown for SED rate and CRP, which come from 93 and 96 individuals, respectively. The changes seen in average values taken in pre- and post- Nutritional Boot Camp tests represent the overall effect of our program. Our results over just a four-week period were simply amazing. Of the 20 measurements we took, we saw statistically true differences in 16 with a confidence level of 99.9%. This is why I feel so confident in The Food Prescription's ability to change people's lives! For more information about our Boot Camp results, see Appendix A.

Weight and BMI

As discussed in Chapter Two, being overweight needs to be considered a chronic illness, and one that is associated with:
- Coronary heart disease
- Type 2 diabetes
- Cancer
- Hypertension
- High cholesterol
- Stroke
- Liver and gallbladder disease
- Sleep apnea and respiratory problems
- Arthritis
- Gynecological problems, such as infertility and abnormal menstrual periods

Being overweight is a serious matter, and I look at a patient's weight and BMI as indicators of their overall health. BMI is calculated as: BMI = Weight (lbs) $\times$ 703 / Height^2 (in^2)

The following standards represent the International Classification of adult weight, according to BMI:
- BMI 18.50 – 24.99 Normal
- BMI 25.00 – 29.99 Overweight
- BMI 30.00 – 39.99 Obese
- BMI > 40 Morbidly Obese

An increase in weight and BMI are two easily measured parameters of underlying metabolic imbalance. Although weight loss is not a sole marker of health improvement, it can be used as a barometer of progress that is easy to measure. Figure 9.1 shows the average weight losses seen by our Boot Camp participants:

Figure 9.1

Weight (in pounds)

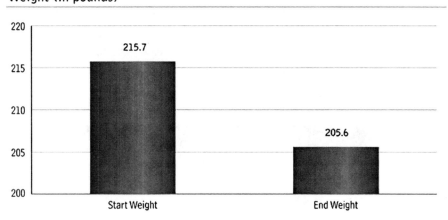

Figure 9.2

BMI

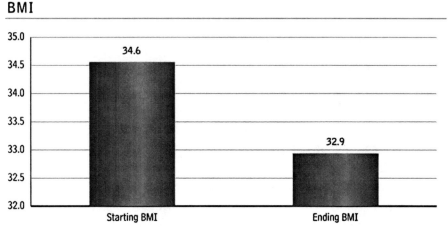

There was an average of 4.7% reduction in weight, from an average baseline weight of 215.74 pounds to an average of 205.61 pounds after nutritional intervention. These findings are of no surprise, as we find weight reduction to be universal in all of our participants who start Boot

Camp with an above normal BMI. It should be noted again that individuals with normal weight and BMI who complete the Boot Camp do not have a significant amount of weight or BMI reduction. However, they do see vast improvements in other health problems, such as high blood pressure or elevated cholesterol. There was an average of 4.7% reduction in BMI, from an average baseline of 34.56 to an average of 32.94 after Boot Camp.

Blood Pressure and Heart Rate

Blood pressure is the force of blood pushing against the walls of arteries. Blood pressure is measured in millimeters of mercury (mm Hg). The classifications in the table below are for people who aren't taking blood pressure-lowering drugs and aren't acutely ill.[1]

Figure 9.3

Category	Systolic (mm Hg)	Qualifier	Diastolic (mm Hg)
Normal	Less than 120	and	Less than 80
Pre-Hypertension	120-139	or	80-89
Stage 1 Hypertension	140-159	or	90-99
Stage 2 Hypertension	160 or higher	or	100 or higher

When a person's systolic and diastolic pressures fall into different categories, the higher category is used to classify blood pressure status. Further, diagnosing high blood pressure is based on the average of two or more readings, taken at each of two or more visits beyond an initial screening.

The heart beats about 60 to 80 times a minute when we're at rest. Technically, a normal heart rate is between 60 and 100 beats per minute. The resting heart rate can increase with normal conditions, such as active exercise or emotional excitement, or abnormal conditions such as dehydration, fever, or poor heart function. The heart rate is able to adapt to changes in the body's need for oxygen, such as during exercise or sleep. It is generally lower in physically fit people and can be a sign of an increased fitness level or better health.2 Here are the results experienced by Boot Camp participants in blood pressure as a result of nutritional intervention over just four weeks: There was an average of 5.5% reduction in SBP and a 3.8% reduction in DBP. These are significant reductions in such a short amount of time. It should be noted that many of these

Figure 9.4

SBP mmHg Systolic Pressure

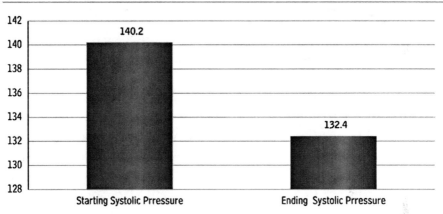

Figure 9.5

DBP mmHg Diastolic Pressure

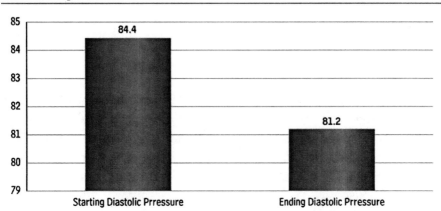

Figure 9.6

Pulse

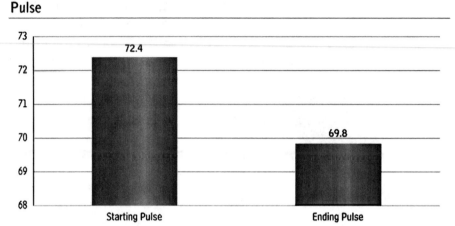

individuals were reducing and discontinuing antihypertensive medications at the same time, making these changes even more impressive.

Change in Heart Rate

There was an average of 3.5% reduction in heart rate. This is quite interesting. Any number of reasons can explain heart rate reduction. I think one explanation with this data set could be due to an increase in volume within the vasculature (blood vessels). In other words, the individuals were better hydrated because of eating all, or mostly, raw fruit and vegetables. Better hydration leads to an improvement in overall circulation, which allows for more efficient heart function. The more efficient the heart functions, the slower it needs to beat.

Inflammation

Inflammation is a process that works to protect the body from infection and foreign substances, like bacteria and viruses. The body's white blood cells and chemicals are sent out to destroy perceived invaders to keep us healthy.[3] This protective force becomes a problem when in some diseases our immune system inappropriately triggers an inflammatory response when there are no foreign substances to fight. These conditions are called autoimmune diseases, which is analogous to "friendly fire." The body has failed to recognize its own constituent parts and causes damage from an immune response against its own cells and tissues.

Inflammation is associated with many chronic diseases, such as diabetes (insulin resistance), anemia, allergies, cancer, heart attack, and more. Below is a list of chronic diseases associated with increased inflammation[4]:

- Allergy
- Alzheimer's
- Anemia
- Aortic valve stenosis
- Arthritis
- Cancer
- Congestive heart failure
- Fibromyalgia
- Fibrosis
- Heart attack
- Kidney failure
- Lupus
- Pancreatitis
- Psoriasis
- Stroke
- Surgical complications

C-reactive protein (CRP) and sedimentation rate (SED Rate) are two blood tests used to measure the amount of inflammation an individual may have. These tests are not specific for any disease type or diagnosis but are useful in assessing the risk an individual has for developing an acute illness, or monitoring an ongoing acute illness. For example, individuals with elevated CRP levels are three times more likely to die from a heart attack than someone with a normal CRP level.[5]

Therefore, we know the higher the CRP level or SED rate level, the greater the risk for developing or worsening a chronic illness. Results experienced by our participants: There was an average of 34.0 % reduction in CRP. The high sensitivity of C-reactive protein (CRP) levels provides a good indicator for inflammation in the circulation system. A reduction in this level is consistent with a reduced amount of inflammation. The amazing thing about these particular findings is that there was a significant reduction of 34% in only four weeks. Furthermore, this reduction occurred in a group of individuals whose baseline values were within the normal range. This likely explains the many reports we hear from our patients and wellness clients of reversal in their arthritis symptoms.

To underscore why a drop of 34% in CRP in such a short time is so exciting, by comparison, a recent trial was done in which a statin drug was shown to decrease CRP. However, it took one year and nine months to show a 37% reduction in CRP.[6] Simply stated, the Nutritional Boot Camp intervention showed a significant antiinflammatory effect faster than the statin drug trial, and within a population that started with CRP levels already within a normal range. Incredible!

There was an average of 31.0% reduction in SED Rate. The SED Rate is a test like CRP that can reveal inflammatory activity in the body. For this test, blood is placed in a test tube and red blood cells will gradually settle to the bottom. If inflammation is present, proteins within the red blood cells will be changed, causing them to clump together. This makes them heavier and they will sink to the bottom of the test tube faster.

Figure 9.7

CRP

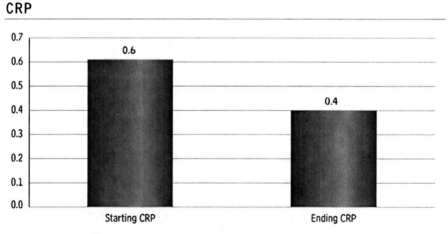

Figure 9.8

SED Rate

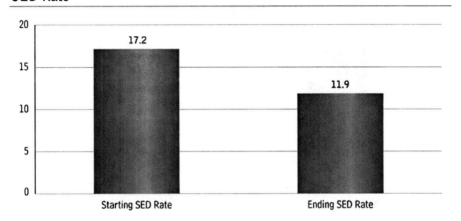

The SED rate test measures the distance red blood cells fall in the test tube within one hour. The further the red blood cells have dropped in that time, the more inflammatories present in the body. A normal range for men is 0-22mm/hour, and for women it is 0-29mm/hour.

Swelling

Swelling is the result of an increase in fluid that is outside of the blood vessels and between the cells of organ tissues. This creates a "puffiness" that is often seen in individuals who are gaining weight. Their weight gain is often due to an increased fluid retention in the body tissues, creating the noticeable puffiness. For Boot Camp, we are able to capture through measurements of the neck and waist, the effects of our program on the reduction of swelling. These measurements are taken immediately before and after nutritional intervention. Here are the results experienced by our participants:

Figure 9.9

Neck (inches)

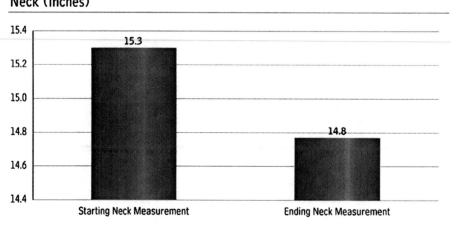

Figure 9.10

Waistline (inches)

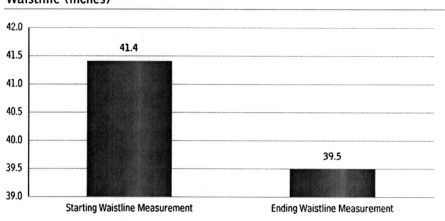

After just four weeks, participants saw an average of 3.5% reduction in the size of their neck circumference and a 4.6% reduction in their waistline measurement. These changes are likely due to a decrease in swelling. We hear universal comments from participants that they see a remarkable decrease in facial swelling as a result of Boot Camp.

Cholesterol

Cholesterol is a waxy, fat-like substance that occurs naturally in all parts of the body. Your body needs some cholesterol to work properly.

But if you have too much in your blood, it can stick to the walls of your arteries. This is called plaque. Plaque can narrow your arteries or even block them. Cholesterol can't dissolve in the bloodstream. It has to be transported to and from the cells by carriers, called lipoproteins. Low-density lipoprotein, or LDL, is known as "bad" cholesterol. High-density lipoprotein, or HDL, is known as "good" cholesterol. These two types of lipids, along with triglycerides and Lipoprotein (a), sometimes called Lp(a) cholesterol, make up your total cholesterol count, which can be determined through a blood test.[7]

Here is how the American Heart Association categorizes total blood cholesterol levels:[8]

Figure 9.11

Total Cholesterol	Category
Less than 200 mg/dL	Desirable
200 to 239 mg/dL	Borderline High
240 mg/dL and above	High Blood Cholesterol

LDL (Bad) Cholesterol. Low-density lipoprotein (LDL) carries cholesterol through the bloodstream and can slowly build up in the inner walls of arteries that feed the heart and brain. Together with other substances, it can form plaque, a thick, hard deposit that can narrow the arteries and make them less flexible. This condition is known as atherosclerosis. If a clot forms and blocks a narrowed artery, a heart attack or stroke can result. LDL blood cholesterol levels are categorized as:

Figure 9.12

LDL Cholesterol Level	Category
Less than 100 mg/dL	Optimal
100 to 129 mg/dL	Near or Above Optimal
130 to 159 mg/dL	Borderline High
160 to 189 mg/dL	High
190 mg/dL and above	Very High

HDL (Good) Cholesterol. Approximately one-fourth to one-third of blood cholesterol is carried by high-density lipoprotein (HDL). HDL cholesterol is known as "good" cholesterol because high levels of HDL seem to protect against heart attack. Low levels of HDL (less than 40 mg/dL) also increase the risk of heart disease. Medical experts think that HDL tends to carry cholesterol away from the arteries and back to the liver, where it's passed from the body. Some experts believe that HDL removes excess cholesterol from arterial plaque, slowing its buildup. HDL blood cholesterol levels are categorized as:

Figure 9.13

HDL Cholesterol Level	Category
Less than 40 mg/dL (Men) Less than 50 mg/dL (Women)	Low HDL. A major risk factor for heart disease
60 mg/dL and above	Protective levels of HDL cholesterol

Triglycerides. Triglyceride is a form of fat made in the body. Elevated triglycerides can be due to being overweight, physically inactive, smoking cigarettes, excess alcohol consumption, or a diet very high in overly processed carbohydrates (60 percent of total calories or more). People with high triglycerides often have a high total cholesterol level, including a high LDL (bad) level and a low HDL (good) level. Many people with heart disease or diabetes also have high triglyceride levels. Triglycerides are categorized as:

Figure 9.14

Triglyceride Level	Category
Less than 150 mg/dL	Normal
150 to 199 mg/dL	Borderline High
200 to 499 mg/dL	High
500 mg/dL and above	Very High

Lipoprotein (a), or Lp(a) is a close cousin of LDL cholesterol. Because of their similarity, tests don't always separate levels of LDL from Lp(a), including both within the LDL measurement. Of interest, medications aimed at reducing high LDL may not achieve desired results, as Lp(a) may be resistant to a particular treatment. Like LDL, Lp(a) is thought to contribute to the buildup of fatty deposits in artery walls.

Figure 9.15

Total Cholesterol

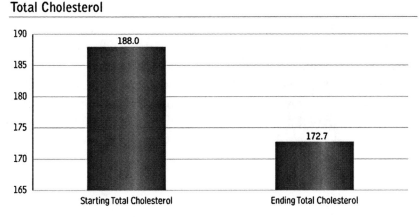

Figure 9.16

LDL

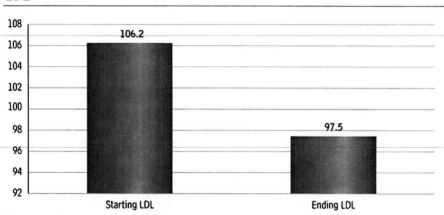

Figure 9.17

HDL

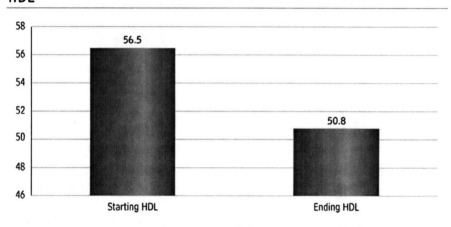

The results of cholesterol decline in our participants, as a result of nutritional intervention were impressive. After just four weeks, there was an across-the-board decrease in cholesterol, with an average of 8.1% reduction in total cholesterol and an 8.3% reduction in LDL. Although we also saw a 10.1% reduction in HDL cholesterol, this change did not affect the overall total cholesterol to HDL cholesterol ratio. Furthermore, it is likely that the reduction in HDL cholesterol seen in individuals following healthy, plant based diets is due to a reduction in demand for HDL cholesterol. The reduction in HDL cholesterol did not adversely affect the total cholesterol to HDL ratio.

Blood Sugar

Blood sugar level is the amount of glucose (sugar) in the blood. It is also known as plasma glucose level. The normal range for a fasting blood sugar is 60 mg/dl, to about 100 g/dl. Glucose comes from carbohydrate foods. It is the main source of energy used by the body. Insulin is a hormone that helps the body's cells use glucose. The pancreas produces insulin and then releases it into the blood when glucose levels rise. When adequate amounts of insulin are available and the body's cells respond to it normally, blood glucose levels remain within the normal range.

When fasting blood glucose levels are above 126 mg/dL, an individual is said to have diabetes. The most common form of the disease is type 2 diabetes, a condition where the body's cells do not respond normally to insulin. Individuals with fasting blood glucose levels between 100 and 125 mg/dL are considered prediabetic. At these levels, the body is experiencing insulin resistance.

Figure 9.18

Glucose

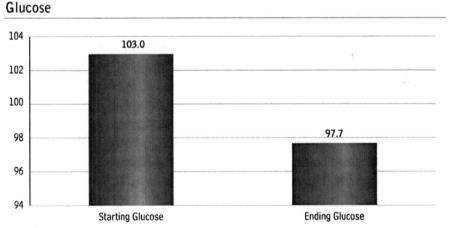

Figure 9.19

Hem A1C

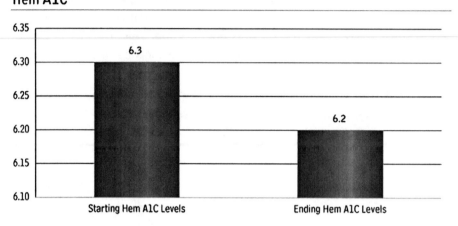

During a four-week nutritional intervention program, our partici-pants experienced, on average, a 5.1% reduction in fasting glucose levels. These findings are impressive, given the fact that many of the partici-pants were diabetics, who were discontinuing insulin and oral diabetic medications at the same time as changing their eating patterns. Another way to evaluate blood sugar levels is through a Hemoglobin A1C test (Hem A1C). This test measures the amount of glucose attached to the hemoglobin molecule of red blood cells, with the result expressed as a percentage. This number gives an indication of the average daily blood sugar levels over a three-month period. Starting in 2010, the American Diabetes Association is recommending A1C tests as a diag-nostic tool for diabetes. Unlike blood glucose testing, the test for A1C doesn't require fasting and can be beneficial for earlier detection of pre-diabetes conditions. 9 A person without diabetes would have an A1C of about 5%. Those with a pre-diabetic condition would have an A1C of 5.7-6.4%.

Individuals with A1C of 6.5% or higher are considered diabetic. For our participants, there was an average of 1.7% reduction in Hem A1C. The significant change in hemoglobin A1C results supports the changes seen in fasting glucose levels.

Kidney Function

Blood urea nitrogen (BUN) and Creatinine are two substances measured in the blood used to assess kidney function.

BUN—Blood urea nitrogen (BUN) measures the amount of urea nitrogen, a waste product of protein metabolism in the blood. Ammonia is a toxic substance that is produced in the liver as a byproduct of certain foods (e.g. animal flesh protein). The liver converts ammonia to urea, which is carried by the blood to the kidneys for excretion. Because the kidneys clear urea from the bloodstream, a test measuring how much urea nitrogen remains in the blood is useful as a test of renal function. The normal level of BUN in adults is 7- 20mg/dL. Values can vary slightly, depending on the lab.[10] However, there are many factors besides renal disease that can cause BUN alterations, including protein breakdown, hydration status, and liver failure.

Figure 9.20

BUN

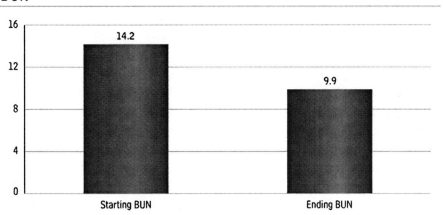

Figure 9.21

Creatinine

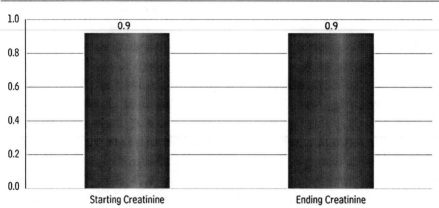

Creatinine—Measuring serum Creatinine is a useful and inexpensive method of evaluating kidney function. Creatinine is a non-protein waste product that is filtered easily when kidneys are operating properly. As the Glomerular Filtration Rate (GFR), or kidney flow rate, decreases, levels of serum Creatinine rise. When tested, if the serum Creatinine level doubles, the GFR is considered to have been halved. A threefold increase is considered to indicate a 75% loss of kidney function.[11]

In measures of kidney function, our participants experienced the above. Over a four-week period, our Boot Camp participants saw, on average, a 30.3% reduction in BUN, and an average 32.9% reduction in BUN/Creatinine ratio. There was no significant reduction in Creatinine. These findings are consistent with an improvement in kidney flow as a result of improved hydration. A high BUN/ Creatinine ratio can be due to dehydration. This ratio decreases as hydration improves within the blood vessels. Increased hydration within the blood vessels allows the heart and vascular system to work more efficiently, and the kidney gets better blood flow.

Figure 9.22

BUN/Creatinine

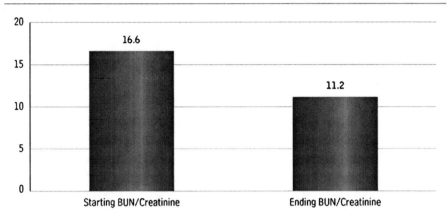

Figure 9.23

CO2

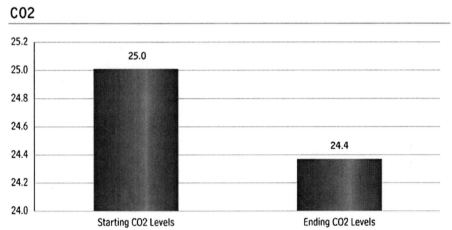

Carbon Dioxide Level (CO2)

There was an average of 2.6% reduction in CO_2 level. Carbon dioxide is a measure of the amount of acid in the bloodstream. It has little meaning within its normal range. However, the significant reduction in the average CO_2 level could be due to an improvement in hydration within the blood vessels. When the body is very dehydrated, CO_2 levels increase due to a decrease in volume within the circulation system.

Summary

In general, we see a universal improvement for people who partici-pate in the Nutritional Boot Camp. Participants experience weight loss along with a reduction in overall body girth, measured as a decrease in neck size and waistline. Additionally, they appear to have better circula-tion because of improved hydration. Biochemically, there is a reduction in cholesterol and blood sugar.

Perhaps most exciting is the significant decrease our participants see in the amount of inflammation they carry in their bodies. This reduction is very important because of the strong association that exists between inflammation and so many chronic diseases, including high blood pres-sure, heart disease, and diabetes. These findings from our Boot Camps support the clinical findings we see in our patients and clients, treated long-term. These findings include the control and reversal of heart dis-ease, chronic lung disease, kidney disease, arthritis, and diabetes.

The Food Prescription of the day is optimal nutrition for optimal health!

౿౿

Chapter Ten
Putting It All Together

> *It is my belief that families pass down diseases more effectively through recipes than through genes. Instead of struggling to untangle lethal genes, we should work to untangle the lethal recipes that are killing us*
>
> **—Baxter D. Montgomery, MD, FACC**

Over the years of promoting the concepts of *The Food Prescription*, I am frequently asked various questions that could be classified under different themes. The *scientific questions* include, "Where do I get my protein?" "What about calcium?" Or "Don't growing children need their meat and milk?" The *entitlement questions* include, "Why can't I have a little chicken occasionally?" Or "Is a small amount of fish acceptable every now and then?" Lastly, the *inheritance questions* include, "How can nutrition control my diabetes if it is in my genes?" Or "Isn't heart disease genetic?" These questions and many more like them are primarily the result of an excess of misinformation transmitted through the general public. Nevertheless, these typical comments and questions represent a much more complex set of issues related to our nation's overall health condition. It has been my goal to address many of these complexities in *The Food Prescription*.

In this concluding chapter, I wish to leave you with some "take home" points to simplify further the concepts discussed in this book and undo much of the confusion and misinformation that exists. My summary approach will be to address the following basic questions:
* What can I eat?
* What about protein?

- What about genetics?
- Do I have to become a vegan or vegetarian?
- What about exercise?

What can I eat?

In March of 2009, I was blessed with the opportunity to speak before a large church congregation in Houston at each of their four weekend worship services. I talked extensively about the ability of the human body to heal itself, but I made it very clear that it required people to remove all animal products and processed foods from their diets. My comments were well received by the congregation, including the pastor and his wife. During a subsequent meeting with the church pastor and his chief financial officer, the question of "What can I eat?" was raised.

This was not the first time I had heard this question. In fact, it was and is a frequently asked question. However, the question resonated in a very different way this time. It finally occurred to me that when one recommends the removal of baked chicken, baked fish, bacon, sausage, cheese, eggs, milk, bread, cereal, etc. from the diet, there appears to be nothing left to eat. It was at this very moment that this question transformed beyond a fundamental question to an immensely profound statement that implied an important concept. This question of "What can I eat?" evolved into the possibilities of "What I can eat and be healthy?" "What I can eat and be satisfied?" "What I can eat and be more vibrant?" "What I can eat and live life more abundantly?" When removed from the familiar, we have an immediate sense of feeling lost. This occurs even when the familiar is harmful to us. Although chicken, fish, eggs, cereal, milk, etc. are bad for us, these foods are what we have been eating all of our lives, and hence bring about a certain sense of safety. This becomes apparent when individuals in our Boot Camp frequently state that removing animal protein, dairy, and processed carbohydrates have helped them, but wonder if it's right to remove these things from their children's diet.

The familiarity of certain foods, determined to be toxic to our bodies, makes it difficult for people to accept fully that these foods should not be eaten by anyone! Closely related to the concept of what can I eat is the question, "Is it okay to eat meat, fish, dairy, eggs, or processed foods some of the time?" I often respond to this question by stating that we live in a free society, and consuming these foods on rare occasion is not against any laws that I know of. Therefore, it is "okay" to eat them. But it is important this statement comes with a disclaimer. We need to accept that these foods are "biochemically" bad for us, and will potentially do harm to our bodies when consumed in any amounts. It is always the best advice to leave these foods out of our diets completely.

I am given many examples of people who eat animal protein, dairy, eggs, and processed foods and are "doing well." There are also examples of individuals who jump from airplanes, who have parachutes that fail to open and live to tell about the experience. I have heard that members of certain religious cults allow rattlesnakes to bite them and live to tell about it. Many things in life are tolerable but not advised. Hence, just as I would advise you not to jump from an airplane with a defective parachute or allow yourself to be bitten by a rattlesnake, I advise you not to eat meat, fish, dairy, eggs, or processed foods.

What about protein?
The question or concern about protein in a plant-based diet is perhaps the most frequent one I get. This is what I would call a scientific-themed question. Other similar questions include "Do I need to take a calcium supplement?" "Do I need to take a multivitamin?" "Is this way of eating beneficial for growing children or pregnant women?" Or "Will I lose too much weight if I am a normal weight to start with?"

Simply stated, consuming plant-based foods that are not overly processed is what the body needs. As stated in the *Nutrition Basics* chapter, the body only needs the essential amino acids in order to make all of the protein it needs. Natural plant-based foods are the best forms of nutrition and therefore are not only good for children and pregnant women, they are essential. Regarding calcium and multivitamins, these substances are best obtained from plant-based foods. The only vitamin supplements that I recommend on occasion are B12 and Vitamin D.

Vitamin B12 deficiency occurs because our living environment is too sanitary, with constant washing of our hands and cleaning ourselves with soaps fortified with antibiotics. As a result, we do not carry the necessary bacterial flora in our bodies for the natural production of Vitamin B12. The best source of Vitamin D is the sun. Many of us have lifestyles that limit our time in the sun, giving us lower levels of Vitamin D. Individuals in this situation may need to supplement their diet with Vitamin D supplements, while trying to increase their sun exposure.

What about genetics?

It is commonly thought that certain diseases such as diabetes, heart disease, cancer, and hypertension are determined solely, or primarily, by genetic predisposition. "Heart disease is very prevalent in my family, so there is nothing I can do," is a common statement I hear. All of our body's functions are controlled by genes, and therefore they are all genetic by definition. This makes all diseases technically genetic in origin as well. It is important to understand that our genes do not necessarily determine *that* we will get sick. They essentially determine *how* we get sick, if we *do* get sick. Our genes have good components and bad components. If exposed to a bad environment, as is the case with bad foods, they express cell products that predispose us to disease states. When exposed to a good environment, such as having access to only good food, they express cell products that allow for optimal health or disease reversal.

For example, if 1,000 individuals ate the very same amount of fried animal protein, dairy, and processed foods regularly, they would all get sick. However, they would get sick in different ways. Some would get fat (likely most), some would develop diabetes and hypertension, some would develop diabetes and heart attacks, and yet others would neither get fat nor develop a common chronic disease, but would become depressed or emotionally unstable.

In essence, *how* they get sick would be determined by their genetics, but *that* they get sick would be determined by the food they eat. Conversely, if the same group of individuals ate a minimally processed, whole food, plant-based nutritional diet, they would all develop the same condition of optimal health, without physical or emotional illness. The same genes that will predispose them to sickness in the setting of bad food will predispose them to optimal health in the setting of good food.

Do I have to become a vegan or vegetarian?

I am not recommending that you become a vegan or vegetarian. I am recommending that you discontinue eating all forms of dead animal flesh, dairy, eggs, processed vegetables, and artificial supplements. These statements may seem contradictory, but they are not. In the grand scheme of things, individuals who consume vegan or vegetarian diets are healthier than individuals who consume diets with animal protein and dairy. However, it is important to apply basic concepts to the food you eat, rather than basic labels. There are many foods that are classified vegetarian, vegan, or even raw vegan, that are unhealthy. It is possible for a vegetarian or vegan to go an entire year (or even a lifetime) without eating a single serving of a fresh fruit or vegetable. The simple concept of healthy eating is to eat natural plant-based foods that are not overly processed. Plant-based foods that are juiced, blended as a smoothie, seasoned whole and raw, lightly steamed, boiled, or slowly warmed, or dehydrated at low heat are generally within the realm of foods that allow for, or promote, optimal health.

The food classification system was designed to give a perspective on the relative health value of food. Ideally, one should eat within Levels 0 to 4. However, an individual who eats at Levels 0 to 4, roughly 95% of the time, and eats a small serving of fish (meeting a Level 7 standard) once every 4 to 6 months, may achieve better health than someone else may, who eats deep fried tofu and rice sautéed in olive oil, daily, but never eats dairy or animal flesh. The person in the second example is technically on a vegan diet, but this individual eats at a Level 10 daily, and by far is eating less healthy than the person is in the first example. Eating plant-based foods is very important; however, what is done to the plants before they are eaten is equally important from a health perspective.

What about Exercise?

When counseling patients or wellness clients on the importance of complying with a nutritionally excellent plan, frequently they ask about exercise. The question posed is, "What about exercise doc?" My response in that case is to say that while exercise is very important, proper nutrition is everything. In the context of overall wellness, it is always important that we nourish our bodies properly. I frequently ask my wellness clients during Boot Camp lectures, if they were to drink a 6-ounce glass of water with cyanide in it, how far would they have to run in order to run it off? The usual response is a set of blank stares, plus or minus a few grimaces. The point is clear that cyanide is a poison, and it is not a matter of running it off, it is a matter of keeping it out of your system.

The same concept applies to poor nutrition. As stated in earlier chapters, there are many aspects of the standard American diet that place it within the category of being toxic or poisonous. The body does not function well when fed poor nutrition. Exercise in this setting may make things worse. So it is important to understand that an optimal exercise program begins with an optimal nutritional program.

There are numerous benefits of exercise that are both independent of, and complementary to, an excellent nutritional program. So, while our focus in this book is nutritional excellence, it is important that we spend some time discussing the importance of exercise, as it relates to overall health and proper nutrition.

Some of the generally known benefits of exercise are listed below.
- Exercise improves your mood. Physical activity stimulates various brain chemicals that may leave you feeling happier and more relaxed, after you work out than before you work out.

Regular exercise can boost your confidence and boost your self-esteem.
- Exercise helps combat chronic disease. Heart disease, osteoporosis, obesity, and diabetes, as well as lipid disorders can be partially controlled with regular exercise. Regular physical activity is known to boost the so-called "good" cholesterol, which is the high-density lipoprotein (HDL), and decrease triglycerides. Regular exercise can also improve insulin sensitivity in type 2 diabetics, and improve bone mass in individuals with osteoporosis. It is also thought to prevent certain types of cancer.
- Exercise can boost your energy level. Individuals who exercise regularly are known to have decreased breathing effort during

routine activities of daily living. The reason for this is that regular exercise allows the heart and lungs to function more efficiently, allowing you to enjoy your activities of daily living with greater ease.

- Exercise promotes better sleep. Routine physical activity during the day has been shown to improve quality and duration of sleep at night. A caveat is that you should not exercise too close to bedtime as this may prevent or delay you from falling asleep.
- Exercise can enhance one's sexual life. Improvement in physical activity can improve one's overall energy, which enhances your sex life. Women are known to have enhanced sexual arousal, and men are known to have fewer problems with erectile dysfunction by participating in regular exercise.

Exercise can be fun, if it is made to be fun. It can also improve overall social interactions with family, friends, and other loved ones.

- Exercise enhances dietary compliance. Researchers have shown that moderate exercise in obese women improved their dietary compliance, thus having a synergistic effect toward enhancing their weight loss.[1]

Exercise has multiple benefits, in many different areas of health. There are numerous physiological benefits of exercise that are beyond the scope of this discussion. Suffice it to say, regular exercise is an important part of one's overall health and wellbeing. The proper amount of exercise in the proper environment, exposed to fresh air and sunlight, is an excellent companion to an excellent nutritional program.

Where Can I Go for Help and Support?

We know that making lifestyle changes can be challenging, and no single approach is right for everyone. That's why the Montgomery Heart and Wellness Center offers different services to meet specific needs. As you take those first steps towards changing your health and life for the better, you can be confident that we are here to help you achieve your goals. Services we provide include:

- In Person Nutritional Boot Camp
- Online Nutritional Boot Camp

- Private, Onsite Wellness Coaching with Dr. Montgomery
- Small groups, Onsite Wellness Coaching with Dr. Montgomery

Summary

I often hear comments about how "extreme" *The Food Prescription* program is. On the surface of things, I understand how an individual might think this way. The food we eat is fully integrated into our lives. Food is associated with our holidays, celebrations, times of mourning, work, recreation, as well as our times of boredom and excitement. Turkey and dressing on Thanksgiving; barbecue for the Fourth of July; pizza with a study group; hotdogs on a campout. These are all examples of how particular foods have become essentially synonymous with various occasions. Following *The Food Prescription* can have an impact on our ability to socialize with friends and family, as special arrangements are occasionally needed when natural plant-based foods are not readily available.

The social impact, though major, is only one aspect of the change. An individual who takes on these changes may have to change the way they buy, store, and prepare their food. For example, someone who eats out regularly may have to limit his or her selection of eateries, or eat out less. They may feel the need to purchase special food preparation tools such as a blender, food processor, or a dehydrator. Also, an increase in cost is often mentioned as a problem because of a perceived need to buy all organic produce. In essence, such changes we think will cause the need to *unravel* our lives. However, if we were to closely evaluate our current national health condition as discussed in Chapters One and Two, we would find that our lives are progressively becoming *unraveled* by our poor health. We regularly suffer from headaches, allergies, mood disorders, insomnia, impotence, loss of libido, fatigue, attention deficit disorder, aches and pain from arthritis, and a generalized decrease in mobility. These common health conditions are often associated with many advanced disease states such as heart disease, cancer, diabetes, and more.

Unfortunately, many of these diseases begin *before* the prime of our lives. Our current solutions to these problems consist of over-the-counter and prescription drugs, artificial vitamins and herbs, invasive medical procedures and surgeries. These forms of medical treatment often result in other problems, such as side effects that often mimic other diseases or worsen the conditions they are used to treat. Not only are we plagued with the side effects of our current "solutions," we are greatly affected by their monetary costs. These common illnesses create a major financial strain on us, individually and nationally.

However, despite the various side effects and costs, the worst aspect of the current forms of health care treatments is that they simply do not result in disease prevention, control, or reversal. In other words, *they don't work!*

While *The Food Prescription* approach seems extreme on the surface, a closer look reveals otherwise. Individuals who follow the program enjoy immediate benefits of improved energy level, achievement of ideal body weight, reduction of medications, and achievement of a more youthful appearance. This approach is effective at every level of health. Athletes trying to improve their fitness and performance levels; young adults with mild test abnormalities; older individuals with severe health conditions, all benefit from this program. The program can be tailored to allow for less stringent approaches for individuals with mild health problems, versus more stringent approaches for the severely ill. All have benefited from *The Food Prescription* approach.

The majority of our wellness clients enjoy the benefits of immediate improvement in their health that is not only sustained over time, but continues to improve. The upfront, aggressive nutritional intervention of *The Food Prescription* is a critical component to its success. The continued educational components are also important, as they empower individuals to become their own health care experts. If we continue in our current approach of trying to find the next "magic bullet" pill, manipulate the next lethal gene, or design the next high tech surgical procedure while ignoring the obvious underlying cause of why we are ill, the problem will only persist. In this setting, we will pass on a legacy of sickness and disease to future generations. Stroke, heart attack, kidney failure, obesity, diabetes, and many other chronic illnesses will be the new normal health conditions of Americans, of all ages. This sad future need not become a reality. The most important aspect of

The Food Prescription is that it represents a simple, definitive solution to halting our current progressive and declining health condition. *The Food Prescription for Better Health* is just what the doctor ordered!

> ### Tell Us What You Think
> *I hope you have found The Food Prescription for Better Health to be both enjoyable and informative reading. I wish to get your feedback on how this book helped you to improve your overall health. I also want to know how I can make future versions of this book, better. Please take a few moments to share your insights by completing a short questionnaire on our website at drbaxtermontgomery.com/online-store/review/ Thank you for your help.*

∽

Appendices
Appendix A

About Dr. Montgomery and Montgomery Heart and Wellness

Dr. Baxter Montgomery's passion for nutrition began in 2002, when his mother died of complications resulting from heart disease and diabetes, and of the medications used to treat these chronic illnesses. He was just 38 and saw that his own cholesterol was higher than ideal. After much research, he realized a healthy diet was plant-based, and animal-based foods had to go. He changed his diet, got his cholesterol down, and began to build nutritional teaching into his practice. Food became a powerful prescription he could write, with the power to restore good health.

Since his own discovery, Dr. Montgomery has been on a mission to help others. Besides routinely counseling patients on the superior nature of a plant-based diet, he has established nutritional bootcamp programs that to date have helped hundreds of his patients and wellness clients, take back control of their own health conditions. His success in changing lives has made him a highly sought out speaker for national radio, television, church, and community organizations. In 2009, he received the prestigious Benjamin Spock Award for Compassion in Medicine from the Physicians Committee for Responsible Medicine (PCRM) for his leadership in promoting healthier living with plant-based diets.

Dr. Montgomery's current and future plans involve expanding his Nutritional Boot Camps to cover larger organizations, such as corporations, fitness groups, small towns, and rural communities. He hopes that these efforts along with his online resources will help stimulate Americans to make the fundamental changes in their health that is critical to their quality of life.

He also plans to change how health care professionals in this country approach treatment of chronic diseases. He offers his prescription for making a difference to other physicians:

> American medicine needs to change its focus. Medical practice has become a process of prescribing medicines and procedures to treat the side effects of the bad foods we eat. The key issue for true health is a healthy lifestyle, and the core of that lifestyle is optimal nutrition. That needs to be the focus of our practice.
>
> **—Baxter D. Montgomery, MD, FACC**

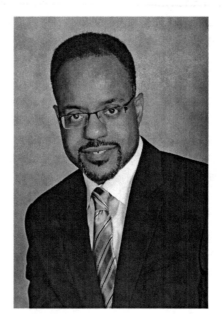

About Dr. Baxter Montgomery

Dr. Baxter Montgomery is a busy cardiologist in Houston, TX. In his private practice, he manages patients with cardiac arrhythmias and coronary heart disease, as well as other chronic illnesses such as hypertension, diabetes, obesity, and inflammatory conditions. He performs a variety of highly technical invasive procedures, such as coronary angiography, cardiac pacemaker and defibrillator implants, electrical catheter ablation for heart arrhythmias, and other hospital procedures. He is the founder and medical director of the Houston Cardiac Association and the Montgomery Heart and Wellness centers, both located near the Texas Medical Center in Houston, Texas. He is a Clinical Assistant Professor of Medicine in the Division of Cardiology at the University of Texas Health Science Center in Houston, and a Fellow of the American College of Cardiology, where he is responsible for teaching doctors who are undergoing subspecialty training in general cardiology and cardiac electrophysiology. Dr. Montgomery is also the founder and executive director of the Johnsie and Aubary Montgomery Institute of Medical Education and Research. Dr. Montgomery enjoys the blessings of his four wonderful children. To learn more about Dr. Montgomery, visit the website (drbaxtermontgomery.com).

Appendix B
Montgomery Heart and Wellness Boot Camp Results

The results listed represent the average values of over 200 individuals who have participated in our Nutritional Boot Camp, with the exception of SED rate and CRP, which represents 93 and 96 individuals, respectively. The changes seen in average values represent the overall effect of the Nutritional Boot Camp intervention.

Data was collected immediately before and after the Nutritional Boot Camp intervention. Of note, most Boot Camp sessions lasted for four weeks. However, three groups had sessions that lasted for five weeks. Hence, our results represent a four to five-week nutritional intervention. The shaded data represents clinical measures that showed a statistically significant change from before and after the nutritional Boot Camp. As you can see, every factor except for three had substantial improvement in just four weeks! See our actual data on the following page:

Nutritional Boot Camp Results

Name	Variable	Mean Baseline	Mean Final	Net Change	Footnote
Weight (lbs)	Weight	215.74	205.61	-10.13	n = 209, t = -26.41, p < 0.001
BMI (kg/ht²)	BMI	34.56	32.94	-1.62	n = 206, t = -26.89, p < 0.001
SBP mmHg	Systolic Pressure	140.20	132.42	-7.78	n = 207, t = -6.15, p < 0.001
DBP mmHg	Diastolic Pressure	84.43	81.20	-3.23	n = 207, t = -5.45, p < 0.001
Heart Rate (bpm)	Pulse	72.39	69.84	-2.55	n = 207, t = -3.28, p < 0.001
Neck Circumference (in)	Neck (inches)	15.30	14.77	-0.53	n = 182, t = -9.16, p < 0.001
Waist Circumference (in)	Waist (inches)	41.41	39.50	-1.91	n = 200, t = -14.53, p < 0.001
Total Cholesteral	Total Cholesteral	187.97	172.75	-15.22	n = 214, t = -7.16, p < 0.001
Triglycerides	Triglycerides	127.16	122.09	-5.07	n = 215, t = -1.1, p = 0.27
HDL	HDL	56.48	50.79	-5.69	n = 214, t = -8.93, p < 0.001

Nutritional Boot Camp Results (continued)

Name	Variable	Mean Baseline	Mean Final	Net Change	Footnote
LDL	LDL	106.24	97.47	-8.77	$n = 210$, $t = -5.13$, $p < 0.001$
Cholesterol HDLC Ratio	Chol/HDLC Ratio	3.55	3.59	0.04	$n = 212$, $t = 0.77$, $p = 0.44$
Glucose	Glucose	102.97	97.68	-5.29	$n = 215$, $t = -218$, $p = 0.03$
BUN	BUN	14.17	9.88	-4.29	$n = 214$, $t = -12.25$, $p < 0.001$
Creatinine	Creatinine	0.92	0.92	0.00	$n = 215$, $t = 0.14$, $p = 0.89$
BUN Creatinine Ratio	BUN/Creatinine	16.62	11.16	-5.46	$n = 205$, $t = -7.85$, $p < 0.001$
C-Reactive Protein Levels (mg/liter)	CRP	0.61	0.40	-0.21	$n = 96$, $t = -5.13$, $p < 0.001$
SED Rate	SED Rate	17.17	11.85	-5.32	$n = 93$, $t = -3.38$, $p < 0.001$
CO2	CO2	25.01	24.37	-0.64	$n = 214$, $t = -3.81$, $p < 0.001$
Hemoglobin A1C	Hem A1C	6.29	6.18	-0.11	$n = 203$, $t = -2.88$, $p < 0.001$

Paired t tests were used to compare the initial and five-week measures. Only subjects that had both an initial and a five-week value were included in the analysis. There were 368 subjects in the program. The n on the graph reports the number of pairs where data was available.

∽

Appendix C
Recipes for Nutritional Detoxification

Early Morning Hydration Protocol— Drink at least 16oz to 32oz of one of the following recommended beverages shortly after waking in the morning:

Water
- Filtered Tap Water
- Bottle Water with a pH of >/= 7.0 (glass bottle preferable)

Apple Cider Vinegar-aide
- 1 cup Agave Nectar
- 1 cup Apple cider Vinegar
- 64 ounces filtered water
- Fresh mint to taste
- Combine all ingredients and mix well

Raw Lemonade or Limeade
- 15 ounces of fresh squeezed lemon or lime juice (must be unpasteurized)
- 1 to 1 ½ of Agave Nectar
- 3 quarts of water
- Mix ingredients then dilute to one gallon

Recommended Power Shots

Apple Cider Vinegar (ACV) Shots
- 2 ounces of unpasteurized ACV
- 1 ounce of raw Agave Nectar
- Mix together. This mixture can be drank multiple times daily, or added to seasoning and used as a salad dressing.

E3 Live® Shots
- 2 ounces of blue green algae (E3-Live Live®)
- I ounce of raw Agave Nectar
- Mix together

Recommended Power Smoothies

Kale Power Smoothie—Kale, Blueberries, Strawberries & E3 Live®
- 2 cups of pure water
- 4 cups of kale
- 2 cups of blueberries
- I cup of strawberries
- 3 dates, soaked
- 2 ounces of E3 Live®
- Blend all ingredients in a Vita Mix blender or other high speed blender until smooth
- Prep time: 10 minutes
- Yield: I serving

Spinach Power Smoothie—Spinach, Pineapple, Mango and Banana
- 2 cups of pure water
- 4 cups of spinach
- 2 medium bananas, frozen
- I mango
- 1.5 cups of pineapple
- 2 ounces E3 Live®
- Blend all ingredients in a high speed blender until smooth
- Prep time: 10 minutes
- Yield: I serving

Flax Hemp Power Shake
- Use water as liquid medium
- Hemp seed protein powder
- Use ½ cup of Agave Nectar as sweetener (add more or less for desired sweetness)
- 1-2 cups of one or more of the following fruits (frozen): pine-apples, blueberries, raspberries, blackberries, pomegranate seeds, strawberries or peaches.
- Two ounces of E3 Live®

- One tablespoon of whole flax seeds (grind with coffee grinder before mixing)
- Add ice as desired for texture. (Optional)

Recommended Super Green Meals

Generic Super Green Meal—Options for Main Component of Super Green Meal
- Organic Spring Mix Greens
- Organic Baby Spinach Greens
- Organic Arugula Greens
- Organic Mache Greens
- Organic Green Sprout Mix

Suggested Additives
- Raisins
- Fresh avocado slices
- Fresh Fruit of choice
- Fresh shredded root vegetables (carrots, beets, raw sweet potatoes, etc.)
- Fresh or dried herb seasonings—Sea Vegetable Seasonings (Sea Seasonings Organic Dulse or Kelp Granules). This is highly recommended!

Suggested Generic Salad Dressing Mix
- One ground avocado slices
- One part vinegar (raw, or unfiltered apple cider vinegar is best, a good balsamic vinegar is good also), lemon juice or lime juice
- One part agave nectar or raw organic honey
- Add water for desired consistency These ingredients can be mixed in a blender with fresh or dried herbs, a small amount of salad greens, a pinch of sea salt, sun dried tomatoes, and/or fruit.

Custom Super Green Meals

Kale Salad
- 5 cups kale
- ½ thinly sliced red onion

- ½ cup chopped red bell peppers
- 1 cup grated sweet potato
- 1 tsp. minced garlic
- 1 tsp. grated ginger root
- 1 tbsp. agave nectar
- ½ cup lemon juice
- 2 tbsp. Braggs Liquid Amino's
- ¼ tsp sea salt

Wash kale and tear into small pieces, removing large stems. Combine all ingredients and toss. Let stand at room temperature for 1-2 hours. Toss again before serving.
Prep Time: 10 minutes—*Yield 6 servings*

Seaweed Salad
- ½ cup hijiki
- ½ cup dulse
- ½ cup wakame
- ¼ tbsp. each orange, yellow and bell pepper
- 1 pkg. Spring salad mix
- 2 Nori sheets, shredded

Hydrate hijiki in a bowl with ½ cup of water. Place the spring salad mix in a large bowl. Add the dulse, wakame, drain the hijiki and add o the salad. Add a pinch of cayenne if you want to add a little spice.
Prep Time: 10 minutes—*Yield 1 serving*

Hijiki & Sprouts
- 1 cup hijiki, soaked
- 1 cup bean sprouts
- 2 tsp lemon juice
- 1 tbsp. dulse seasoning
- 1 tsp tamari or liquid aminos
- ¼ tsp cayenne or red chili pepper
- 2 tsp agave nectar, optional
- ½ cup chopped scallions
- ½ cup diced red peppers

Place the hijiki in a small bowl and soak in lemon juice while you are preparing the other ingredients. Combine all ingredients together, including the hijiki tamari and agave nectar. Toss well and taste. Add more seasonings if needed.

Part II: Recipes for
Nutritional Maintenance

RAW Corn Chips
- 6 ears or 6 cups of corn
- 1 oz cumin
- 1 oz salt
- 1/4 cup flax meal (optional)

Cut the corn to remove the kernels if necessary. Place kernels into a food processor and blend until most of the chunks are gone. Add the salt, cumin and flax. Combine and blend. "Pre-heat" dehydrator at 115 degrees and turn down to 105 degrees when ready to use. Spread the mixture onto a Teflex sheet or solid plastic sheet and place inside of dehydrator. After about 20 minutes, sprinkle some salt and seasonings (optional) across the top. Keep dehydrating until nice and crisp, about 24 hours.

Raw Spinach Dip Recipe
- 2 cups raw baby spinach
- 1 cup raw tahini
- 1 teaspoon sea salt
- 4 cloves of Garlic
- 1 cup filtered water (used only to blend product and thin if necessary)
- 1/2 teaspoon nutmeg (optional)

Combine all ingredients in a food processor and puree.

Corn salad
- 2 cups corn kernels
- ¼ cup red bell pepper, small diced

- ½ cup red onion, small diced
- ½ cup scallions, minced
- ¼ cup cilantro, chopped
- 5 ripe olives, chopped
- 2 tablespoon lemon juice
- 2 oz Braggs liquid aminos
- 2 tbsp ground cumin

Carefully combine all ingredients until well blended. Adjust seasonings to taste and chill.

Guacamole (Regular and Spiced for warmth) 8 servings
- 12 ripe Haas Avocados
- 4 Roma Tomatoes (Seeded and diced)
- 2 c. sweet corn kernels
- 1 bunch Cilantro
- 4 Limes, juiced
- (4 Jalapenos-Spicy only, omit for "regular")
- (1 teaspoon Cayenne Pepper-Spicy only, omit for "regular")

Mix avocado and juice of limes into a paste using masher, blender or food processor. Add tomatoes, corn, chopped cilantro and season to taste with Celtic Sea Salt.

Brownie with icing
- 2 c. dates, soaked
- 1 cup carob powder
- 1 cup cacao powder
- 1/8 cup RAW Tahini paste
- 1 TBSP RAW Agave nectar

A little water may be added if more moisture is needed.
<u>Blend</u> until fully incorporated and mixed together, divide and mold into 6 brownies on a cookie sheet.

Icing:
- 3 avocados
- ½ cup agave nectar

- ¼ cup cocoa powder
- I oz. tahini paste
- I tablespoon vanilla extract
- I tsp salt

METHOD:

Put all ingredients into vita mix blender, and blend on high until smooth and fully incorporated. Spread icing over brownies and leave to set in freezer for I hour.

Key lime Pie
4 servings

Crust:
- ½ cup raw, organic Buckwheat
- ½ cup raw, organic Groats
- 4 Medjool dates
- I tbsp ground golden flaxseed
- 3 tbsp raw agave nectar
- I tsp pink Himalayan sea salt
- ½ tsp of cinnamon
- ½ tsp of nutmeg

Blend all ingredients together in a food proceesor until crust comes together and is fully incorporated. Press evenly into a pie pan covering bottom and insides of inner plate.

Filling:
- 3 large haas avocados
- I large young coconut (use extracted meat)
- I oz young coconut water (use water from coconut)
- 6 large limes (juice and zest)
- ½ cup of agave nectar (sweeten to taste)
- Dash of sea salt

For filling, in food processor or high-speed blender, process all ingre- dients except for one lime's zest. Once smooth and creamy, pour over crust and top with remaining reserved lime zest. Place pie in freezer for 3 hours or until set. Allow to thaw slightly before serving.

Oatmeal Raisin Cookies
- I tbsp ground cinnamon
- I tbsp grated nutmeg
- I tbsp vanilla extract
- I TBSP RAW Agave Nectar
- I cup Raisins
- 2 cups Raw, Organic Groats or Steel Mill Raw Oats
- 8 bananas

Blend all ingredients except raisins, in a blender or food processor until completely combined. Carefully fold together blended ingredients with raisins until fully incorporated. Spoon onto plastic sheet and place into a dehydrator warmed to 105 degrees for 24 hours. Remove when finished and let cool.

5&3 Pasta 4 servings
For the topping:
- I oz Chinese 5 spice
- ½ c Tamari or Nama Shoyu
- I c Shiitake Mushroom
- I Baby Bok Choy; quartered

Add all ingredients together and marinate atleast 30 minutes.

For the "pasta":
- 2 oz spiraled carrot
- 2 oz spiraled Daikon
- 2 oz spiraled Zucchini

Pasta Sauce:
- ½ cup Raw Apple Cider Vinegar
- ½ cup Raw Agave Nectar
- I tsp fresh ginger (root), minced
- I glove garlic, minced

Combine all "Pasta Sauce" ingredients together and toss in the "Pasta" until well coated. Let marinate for 3-5 minutes. Drain excess "sauce" and top with marinated topping.

Marinara Zuchetti
4 servings

Marinara Sauce:
- 3 C fresh Roma Tomatoes
- 20 Sundried Tomatoes, Soaked
- 4 cloves garlic
- 2 cups dates, pitted and soaked
- 2 oz. parsley
- 1 tsp cayenne
- 1 tsp sea salt

Place ingredients in food processor and blend until smooth

Spiral 4 oz. of Fresh Zucchini
Top with Marinara

Sauces and Dressings

Ketchup:
- 4 c. Sun Dried Tomatoes
- 1 ½ c. Apple Cider Vinegar
- ½ c. RAW Agave Nectar
- 2 c. filtered water
- 1 T Ground Mustard

Blend all ingredients until forms thick uniform puree.

Raw Relish:
- 2 English Cucumbers, small to medium dice
- 1 small red onion, same dice as cucumbers
- 1 TBSP Chinese 5 spice
- 1 c Agave Nectar
- ¼ c RAW Apple Cider Vinegar

Combine all ingredients together and store in a container. Acid in vinegar will "break down" and "cook" the relish naturally, after 12-24 hours consistency will be more of a "relish" texture, but just as flavorful and great to use immediately.

Raw Vegan Mustard Recipe
- 1 C yellow mustard, ground
- 1 C apple cider vinegar
- 1 C dates (well packed)
- 2 oz Light agave nectar
- 1 C water
- 2 tsp salt

Combine all ingredients in a blender and blend until creamy, adding water as needed. The mustard may taste quite bitter at first; the bitterness will subside the longer it sits. It is best to make this mustard two or three days before you are planning on using it to let the flavors settle. Store in a jar in the refrigerator for up to two months.

Makes about 3 cups

Strawberry Vinaigrette
- 2 c. frozen strawberries
- 1 c raw agave nectar
- 1 c raw Apple Cider Vinegar
- 2 c filtered water for thinning and taste adjustment
- 1 tsp ground mustard

Blend ingredients together and adjust to taste.

*For the peach dressing, simply replace the strawberries with peaches.

Herbes de Provence Dressing
- 1 oz Herbes de Provence
- 1 tbsp ground mustard
- 4 cloves fresh garlic, minced
- 2 c Raw Agave Nectar
- 2 c Raw Apple Cider Vinegar

Blend ingredients together and adjust to taste.

Smoothies, Juices and Beverages

Green Power Smoothie
- 1 cup Frozen mixed berries
- 1 cup Frozen Strawberries
- 1 cup Fresh kale
- 1 TBSP E-3 live
- 2 cups water (filtered)
- 2 oz. RAW Agave Nectar

In a blender mix all the ingredients until smoothie is blended to desired texture.

Green Power Super Charged Smoothie
- 1 cup Frozen mixed berries
- 1 cup Frozen Strawberries
- 2 cups Fresh kale
- 2 TBSP E-3 live
- 2 cups water (filtered)
- 2 oz. RAW Agave Nectar (or more to taste)

In a blender mix all ingredients until smoothie is blended to desired texture.

Banana Strawberry Smoothie
- 2 cups Frozen Strawberries
- 2 Frozen bananas
- 2 cups water (filtered)
- 2 oz. RAW agave nectar

In a blender mix all ingredients until smoothie is blended to desired texture.

Strawberry Peach Smoothie
- 1 cup Frozen Strawberries
- 1 cup Frozen Peaches
- 2 cups water (filtered)
- 2 oz. RAW agave nectar

In a blender mix all ingredients until smoothie is blended to desired texture.

Pineapple-Cactus Pear Smoothie
- 1 cup Frozen Pineapple Chunks
- 1 cup of Cactus Pear (aka Tuna or Prickly Pear) skinned and seeds removed if desired
- ½ cup Nopal Cactus Paddle, thorns removed and cleaned
- 2 cups filtered water
- 2 oz RAW agave nectar

In a blender mix all ingredients until smoothie is blended to desired texture.

Very Berry Smoothie
- 1 cup Frozen mixed berries
- 1 cup Frozen Strawberries
- 2 cups water (filtered)
- 2 oz. RAW Agave Nectar (or more to taste)

In a blender mix all ingredients until smoothie is blended to desired texture.

Ginger Tea
- 1 ½ –2 inch piece of Fresh Ginger Root, chopped
- 8 oz fresh, filtered water warmed
- 1 TBSP or more Raw Agave Nectar (to taste)

Steep chopped ginger root in water until intensity desired and sweeten to taste with RAW Agave Nectar.

Chamomile Tea
- 1 bag of Chamomile Tea
- 8 oz. warm, filtered water
- 1-2 TBSP Raw Agave Nectar (to taste)

Steep chamomile in warm water until reached desired strength and add agave nectar to sweeten.

RAW Lemonade
- ½ to 1 cup RAW Agave Nectar (Sweeten to taste)
- 1 cup fresh lemon juice
- 4 cups cold water (to dilute)

Blend ingredients well, chill and enjoy!

Soup

Raw tomato soup with Basil

4 servings
- 4 fresh tomatoes
- 3 sun dried tomatoes, soaked in water
- 1 cup basil
- ¼ tsp sea salt

Place all ingredients in the blender and blend until smooth.

Spicy Chili

4 serving
- 2 cups Roma tomatoes
- 4 cups sun dried tomatoes
- 1-2 cloves of garlic or more to taste
- 1 cup Medjool dates
- 1 cup chopped red bell pepper
- 2 teaspoon chili powder
- 1 tablespoon cumin
- 1 tablespoon of cilantro
- Sea salt to taste

Chopped-carrots, celery, red pepper, cilantro, onion, corn Soak sun dried tomatoes in water Drain water from the sun dried tomatoes and blend Add the Roma tomatoes, garlic, dates, bell pepper, Chili powder, cumin, cilantro, and salt into the food processor, and blend until smooth Add chopped celery, red pepper, cilantro, onion, and corn and mix well

Poblano Corn Chowder
- I poblano pepper, seeded and diced
- I medium onion, diced
- 4 cloves garlic, sliced
- 5 c corn
- I c coconut water
- I avocado
- Celtic Sea salt TT

Blend all ingredients, except corn until smooth. Add corn and blend until mostly blended but still slightly chunky.

Wraps
Coconut Wrap "bread"

- 4 c young Thai coconut flesh
- 2 c water
- I t Agave Nectar
- 2T Psyllium Husk
- Seasoning of your choice

Blend all ingredients except Psyllium husk together until creamy. Add Psyllium husk and blend until mixture congeals. Spread thin and dehydrate 110 degrees for 6 hours. Wrap will be dry but pliable.

Baby Spinach Portobello

Avocado Aioli
- Avocado
- Tahini
- Garlic

Marinade for Portobello
- Balsamic vinegar
- Garlic
- Rosemary
- Agave

Place aioli on wrap, top with baby spinach and marinated Portobello mushroom cap sliced on bias.

Tahini Spinach Wrap
- Tahini paste
- Baby spinach
- Thin sliced fennel
- Red bell pepper strips

Zucchini Cremini Mushroom Wrap
- Mixed baby greens
- Zucchini slices
- Quartered cremini mushrooms, topped with "marinara"

Kale leaf wraps
- Carrots
- Cucumber
- Bean sprout
- Avocado
- Ponzu dipping sauce

"Raw" Ponzu dipping sauce
- Juice of I orange, I lime, I grapefruit
- I cup Tamari or Nama Shoyu (Soy Sauce)
- I tsp. Minced Garlic or Garlic Powder
- I tsp. minced ginger

ᘛᘚ

Appendix D
A Few Words from Our Wellness Clients

"I am so pleased to have had a normal cholesterol reading. My cholesterol has always been from mid 200's to high 200's. Only after 12 days on the programs, my cholesterol was in the 180's.

This was my final chance to see if my cholesterol readings could be normal before giving in to taking medication. But what a surprise to know, that by learning about the negative effects of food we consume plays a major part in cholesterol and by changing the types of food to plant base, cholesterol can be lowered.

Thank you Dr Montgomery for seeking another way, a natural way to reversing disease and better health other than manufactured pills"
V.P.

"Dr Montgomery has changed my life by taking time to explain to me the cause of my high blood pressure which he help me lower my BP without medications.

Thanks for I feel much better now and I lost about 30 lbs without working my butt off at the gym"
R.S.

"Now that I have completed the boot camp, I feel much more informed as to what healthy eating really can do for an individual. I went into this expecting to be told I would have limitations on everything that I ate. Not long after that I found that as long as I stayed on course, I could eat as often and as much as I likes. I am now very conscious of what I eat. I still struggle with it at times, but it seems to be getting easier with time.

I no longer have all the junk food cravings. And I laugh every time my coworkers order out for lunch because I know that if I stay focused I will be around a lot longer than I would have had I not changed my

habits. I thank you so much Dr Montgomery and look forward to pressing forward and continuing you maintenance program."
M.M.

"The program worked great! When I started the program, I was taking two blood pressure pills and a pill for high cholesterol. After one week of eating plant based meals, mainly in juice form (pineapple, oranges, apples, celery, grapes, etc.), my blood pressure dropped to normal and I stopped taking both blood pressure pills. The next week I was able to drop the cholesterol pill. My energy is through the roof. Also, the first week, I lost 9 pounds (without any extra exercise). I lost 18 pounds overall in the 4 weeks. I would highly recommend the HCA Wellness program!"
J. O. M.

"Your (Dr. Montgomery) input at every session was very encouraging. The nutritionist was very helpful with her instruction and the food was very tasty also. This several weeks has greatly improved my confidence in improving my health (so simple). I have better overall performance, great energy, no joint pain, no sinus problems, no indigestion, great sleeping and I am sure my blood pressure and glucose levels have improved sizably. I give it an A+."
R.F

"The program has been very informative and helpful. My reason for joining the program was to get off my hypertension medication and that goal has been reached. I have and will continue to recommend this program to family, friends, and colleagues."
C. J-S.

"Wow! Off my diabetes and hypertension medications in two short weeks. This is an incredible program. Thank you for giving me back control of my health and my life."
S.

"This program was fun! The idea of challenging myself every day to stick to the plan was very exciting! I did start to crave foods like rice, shrimp and eggs for some reason, but I was never really hungry. I enjoyed watch-

ing my blood pressure improve. I have and will continue to recommend this program to family and friends."
E.D.

"I thought the program was challenging but rewarding at the same time. It really taught me to focus on more things besides food and I think that everyone should try it. I was also happy with my weight loss and how to have more self control."
S.F.

"I think this is a very good program. It takes a little time to get use to the regiment, but once you get started you realize the changes your body makes. The food you thought you couldn't do without, you can. The body don't crave for things (food) as much. I have not eaten bread or meat for about six weeks. The more you learn about the different foods and how it affects your health, the easier it becomes. Knowledge is power. The body is your temple and we don't realize how we misuse it."
G.F.

"Before starting this program, I would have classified my health between fair and poor. My energy level was quite low. I had difficulty kneeling down to the carpet to clean or play with my grandchild. I always felt tired and sleepy about mid-morning and mid-afternoon. After playing racquetball or any type of exercise, I cold feel my sugar level drop dramatically which resulted in over eating carbs such as bread. But now, I am always full of energy. I can bend down to clean. I can sit on the carpet and play with my grandchild. I can run around the racquetball court without my sugar dropping. I see a difference in my skin too. My daughter has commented on how refreshed I look - and this is at the end of the day! She's also commented on how soft my skin looks just after getting up in the morning. And best of all, my granddaughter has commented on how I look like I'm getting smaller - that's a good thing. I love how I feel and it shows."
E.A.

"This program was excellent because it focused on health improvement and not weight loss although the latter was achieved. I learned that what I eat influences my health on a daily basis and over time. As a result, I believe I will always consider whether what I put in my mouth

is contributing to or detracting from my overall health. The fact that I was able to decrease and/or eliminate certain medications as a result of this program further validates its benefits."
B.D.

"This "wellness" approach is true "healthcare", not "sick care". When people understand how adulterated the "S.A.D." (Standard American Diet) diet is, then they can take better control of their food choices."
P.S.

"I have been a patient of Dr. Montgomery for a long time and I am amazed at the growth of this program. This program works. I have tried dieting, exercise, weight trainers, fasting and on and on. This program put it all together for me and has helped me make it work for a lifetime. Thank you Dr. Montgomery."
R.S.

"Program is Excellent. It has Immediately changed my health and attitude. It makes me work harder at improving MY health. THANK YOU! Highly Recommended."
R.B.

"When I started the program I was on nine different medications. Today I am only on three and will probably get off one more soon. I had very poor sleeping and energy. I sleep about six hours straight and energy level is good. I'm not as tired like I use to be. Blood sugar came down. Blood pressure is better. I lost about 16 pounds. The food is healthy and my appearance is better also. My brothers and sister said you look like your old self. I thank Dr. Montgomery for the information and his good example to all of us who attended the program. I take one step at a time and a full recovery soon. Thanks so much!"
C.C.

"I feel like the new approach to health that I've been taught and the way it was presented to me is going to extend my life. And I find I know I can live with this."
L.H.

I finished treatment for cancer being on chemo, radiation and a new drug, Herciptin, two years ago. Since that time I have only gotten sicker. I could not tolerate any vitamins so with my stress and not eating enough fruits and vegetables. Not even the top Neurologist at MD Anderson could give me enough meds for my migraines. I have not had a migraine in over three weeks now. My energy level is getting better. I am even feeling ready to get back to the gym. My family is very supportive because they are seeing the improvement. This is my new way of life.

V.R.

Appendix E
Resources

For more information on how to improve your health and enhance your life, logon to Dr. Montgomery's website. You can also call our office for information about our various health and wellness services, designed for individuals who live in the Houston area, or are willing to travel. Available services at Montgomery Heart and Wellness:

- **In Person Nutritional Boot Camp**—An intensive program conducted at our Wellness Center, designed to optimize your health and detoxify your body. http://www.drbaxtermontgomery.com/programs/nutritional-boot-camp

- **Online Nutritional Boot Camp**—The same intensive program that is done onsite, completed by participants online. http://www.drbaxtermontgomery.com/programs/nutritional-boot-camp

- **Private, Onsite Wellness Coaching with Dr. Montgomery**—One-on-one, individualized health advice. http://www.drbaxtermontgomery.com/programs/on-site-coaching

- **Private, Phone Wellness Coaching with Dr. Montgomery**—Health advice provided with a phone consultation with Dr. Montgomery at scheduled times. http://www.drbaxtermontgomery.com/programs/phone-coaching

- **Small Group, Onsite Wellness Coaching with Dr. Montgomery**—Groups of two to six participants allow us to tailor our discussions and presentations to meet the specific needs of the group. http://www.drbaxtermontgomery.com/programs/on-site-coaching

- **Online Store Coming Soon**—A variety of materials are available to help make your wellness journey easier.

These sessions are not intended to be a substitute for formal medical advice, or medical care of any type.

Montgomery Heart and Wellness
10480 Main St.
Houston, Texas 77025
Phone Number: 713-599-1144
Fax: 713-599-1199

End Notes

Chapter One

1 World Health Organization. *The World Health Report 2002*. Geneva, Switzerland. 2002. Accessed www.who.int/whr/200/en. Accessed 07/29/10.

2 World Health Organization. "Obesity and Overweight Fact Sheet." September 2006. http:// www.who.int/mediacentre/factsheets/fs311/en/. Accessed 10/14/10.

3 World Health Organization. "10 Facts on Obesity." February 2010. http://www.who.int/features/ factfiles/obesity/en/. Accessed 10/14/10.

4 Grady, Denise. "First Signs of Puberty Seen in Younger Girls." *The New York Times*, August 9, 2010. http://nytimes.com/2010/08/09/health/research/09puberty.html. Accessed 08/26/10.

5 Rautalahti M, Albanes D, Virtamo J, et al. "Lifetime menstrual activity—Indicator of breast cancer risk." *European Journal of Epidemiology*. Vol. 9, No. 1, 17-25. Jan. 1993.

6 Krieger E, Youngaman LD, and Campbell TC. "The modulation of aflatoxin (AFB1) induced preneoplastic lesions by dietary protein and voluntary exercise in Fisher 344 rats." *The FASEB Journal*. 2 (1988): 3304 Abs

7 Xu J M.D., Kochanek K M.A., Murphy S B.S., et al. "Deaths: Final Data for 2007." CDC Division of Vital Statistics. *National Vital Statistics Reports*. Vol. 58, No. 19. Pg 13-14. May 2010. www.cdc.gov/NCHS/data/nvsr/nvsr58/nvsr58_19.pdf. Accessed 09/01/10.

8 American Heart Association. "Cardiovascular Disease Statistics." 2006. http://americanheart.org/ presenter.jhtml?identifier=4478. Accessed 08/17/10.

9 Marchione, Marilynn. "No cure for heart disease, Bill Clinton's case shows." *USA Today*. http:// www.usatoday.com/news/health/2010-02-12-clinton-heart_N.htm. Accessed 08/17/10.

10 Sternberg, Steve. "Russert's death shows heart attack isn't easy to predict." *USA Today*. http://www.usatoday.com/news/health/2008-06-15-heart-attack-russert_N.htm. Accessed 08/17/10.

11 Enos WE, Holmes RH, and Beyer J. "Coronary disease among United States soldiers killed in action in Korea." *JAMA. 1953*,152: 1090-1093.

12 McGill HC Jr, McMahan CA. "Determinants of atherosclerosis in the young. Pathobiological Determinants of Atherosclerosis in Youth (PDAY) Research Group." *American Journal of Cardiology.* 1998 Nov 26;82(10B):30T-36T.

13 Joseph A, Ackerman D, Talley JD, et al. "Manifestations of coronary atherosclerosis in young trauma victims—an autopsy report." Department of Medicine, University of Louisville, Kentucky. *Journal of the American College of Cardiology.* 1993 Aug: 22(2):459-67.

14 National Lung Cancer Partnership. "Lung Cancer in the United States: Facts." 2009. http:// www.nationallungcancerpartnership.org/index.cfm?page=lung_cancer_facts_US. Accessed 8/31/10.

15 Unknown. "Dana Reeve dies of lung cancer at 44." CNN.com. www.cnn.com/2006/SHOWBIZ/03/07/reeve.obit/index.html. Accessed 05/15/10.

16 Centers for Disease Control and Prevention. "Fast Facts about Colorectal Cancer." www.cdc.gov/ cancer/colorectal/basic_info/facts.htm. Accessed 09/03/10.

17 Susan G. Komen for the Cure® website. "Ambassador Nancy G. Brinker bio." http:// www5.komen.org/Content.aspx?id=6062. Accessed 08/17/10.

18 Centers for Disease Control and Prevention." (Breast Cancer) Fast Facts." http://www.cdc.gov/ cancer/breast/basic_info/fast_facts.htm. Accessed 09/03/10.

19 Backer H M.D., MPH. "Prostate Cancer Screening: Exploring the Debate." *The Permanente Journal.* Vol. 3, No. 3. Fall 1999. http://xnet. kp.org/permanentejournal/fall99pj/prostate.html. Accessed 09/03/10.

20 Centers for Disease Control and Prevention. "(Prostate Cancer) Fast Facts." http:// www.cdc.gov/cancer/prostate/basic_info/fast_facts.htm. Accessed 09/03/10.

Chapter Two
1 Centers for Disease Control and Prevention. "Chronic Diseases. The Power to Prevent, The Call to Control. At a Glance 2009." http://www. cdc.gov/chronicdisease/resources/publications/AAG/pdf/chronic.pdf. Accessed 8/11/10.

2 NationMaster.com. "Health Statistics: Obesity (mostrecent) by country." http://www.nationmaster.com/graph/hea_obe-healthobesity. *OECD Health Data 2005.* Accessed 9/17/10.

3 Center for Disease Control and Prevention. "Obesity: Halting the Epidemic by Making Health Easier: At a Glance 2009." www.cdc.gov/chronicdisease/resources/publications/AAG/obesity.htm. Accessed 08/12/10.

4 Kasper DC, Braunwald E, Fauci A, et al. *Harrison'sPrinciples of Internal Medicine.* New York: The McGraw-Hill Companies, Inc. 2005:16th Edition; pg. 2153.

5 Arthritis Foundation. "Arthritis Prevalence: A Nation in Pain." *News from the Arthritis Foundation.* 2008. http://www.arthritis.org/media/newsroom/media-kits/Arthritis_Prevalence.pdf. Accessed 08/ 15/10.

Chapter Three
1 Tortora G and Anagnostako N. *Principles of Anatomy and Physiology, Sixth Edition.* New York: Harper Collins.1990, pgs 6-7.

Chapter Four
1 Choi H M.D., Dr.P.H. "Purine-Rich Foods and the Risk of Gout in Men." *New England Journal of Medicine. 2004; 350:2520-2521. http://www.nejm. org/toc/nejm/350/24/.* Accessed 08/24/2010.

2 Chang-Claude J, Frentzel-Beyme R, Eilber U. "Mortality pattern of German vegetarians after 11years of followup."*Epidemiology.* 1992: Sep; 3(5): 395-401.

3 Fisher M, Levine PH, Weiner, BH, et al."The effect of vegetarian diets on plasma lipid and platelet levels." *Archives of Internal Medicine.* 1986:146.6. **West RO M.D., MPH, and Hayes OB M.P.H.** "A Comparison between Vegetarians and Nonvegetarians in a Seventh-day Adventist Group." *American Journal of Clinical Nutrition,* Vol. 21, 853-862. The American Society for Clinical Nutrition, Inc. 1968.

4 Hoggan R M.A., and Braly J M.D."How Modern Eating Habits May Contribute to Depression." About.com. http://depression.about.com/cs/diet/a/foodallergies.htm. Accessed 08/24/10. About.com Health's Disease and Condition content is reviewed by the Medical Review Board.

5 Martin, Gary. "You Are What You Eat." http://www.easydietforlife.com/you-are-what-youeat.html. Accessed 08/15/2010.

6 Thorogood M, Mann J, Appleby P, et al."Risk of death from cancer and ischaemic heart disease in meat and non-meat eaters." *British Medical Journal.* 1994;308:1667-70. Phillips RL."Role of lifestyle and dietary habits in risk of cancer among Seventh-Day Adventists." *Cancer Research* (Suppl). 1975;35:3513-22. Campbell TC, Chen J. "Diet and chronic degenerative diseases: Perspectives from China." *American Journal of Clinical Nutrition.* 1994;59:1153S–61S. Esselstyn CB Jr, Ellis SG, Medendorp SV, et al."A strategy to arrest and reverse coronary artery disease: a 5-year longitudinal study of a single physician's practice." *The Journal of Family Practice.* 1995; 41:560-8. Salie F. "Influence of vegetarian food on blood pressure." *Med Klin.* 1930; 26:929-31.

7 Chang-Claude J, Frentzel-Beyme R, Eilber U. "Mortality patterns of German vegetarians after 11 years of follow-up." *Epidemiology.* 1992;3:395-401. Phillips RL."Role of lifestyle and dietary habits in risk of cancer among Seventh-Day Adventists." *Cancer Research* (Suppl). 1975;35:3513-22.

8 Campbell TC, Chen J."Diet and chronic degenerative diseases: Perspectives from China." *American Journal of Clinical Nutrition.* 1994;59:1153S–61S. Esselstyn CB Jr, Ellis SG, Medendorp SV, et al."A strategy to arrest

and reverse coronary artery disease: a 5-year longitudinal study of a single physician's practice." *Journal of Family Practice.*1995;41:560-8. Salie F. "Influence of vegetarian food on blood pressure." *Med Klin.* 1930;26:929-31.

9 Fung T ScD, van Dam R PhD, Hankinson S ScD, et al. "Low-Carbohydrate Diets and All-Cause and Cause-Specific Mortality." *Annals of Internal Medicine Abstract.* September 7, 2010; vol. 153 no. 5 289-298. http://www.annals.org/content/153/5/289.abstract.Accessed 9/24/10.

10 Campbell TC PhD and Campbell TM. *The China Study.* Dallas: BenBella Books. 2006.

11 Fisher M, Levine PH, Weiner, BH, et al. "The effect of vegetarian diets on plasma lipid and platelet levels." *Archives of Internal Medicine.* 1986:146.6.

12 Sacks **FM and Kass EH.** "Low blood pressure in vegetarians: Effects of specific foods and nutrients." *American Journal of Clinical Nutrition.* Vol. 48, 795-800. The American Society for Clinical Nutrition, Inc. 1988.

13 Barnard ND, Scialli AR, Bertron P, et al. "Effectiveness of a low-fat veg-etarian diet in altering serum lipids in healthy premenopausal women." *American Journal of Cardiology.* 2000;85:969-72. Salie F. "Influence of vege-tarian food on blood pressure." *Med Klin.* 1930;26:929-31. Hegsted DM. "Calcium and osteoporosis." *Journal of Nutrition.* 1986;116:2316-9.Nich-olson AS, Sklar M, Barnard ND, et al. "Toward improved management of NIDDM: A randomized, controlled, pilot intervention using a low fat, vegetarian diet." *Preventative Medicine.* 1999;29:87-91. Strip C, Overhand K, Christensen J, et al. "Fish intake is positively associated with breast cancer incidence rate." *Journal of Nutrition.* 2003; 133(11):3664-3669. Gellar E, Sans-Gallardo I, Van's Veer P, et al. "Mercury, fish oils, and the risk of myocardial infarction." *New England Journal of Medicine.* 2002; 347:1747-1754.

14 Ismail A., Lee WY. "Influence of cooking practice on antioxidant prop-erties and phenolic content of selected vegetables." *Asia Pacific Journal of Clinical Nutrition.* 2004; 13(Suppl):S162. Barros L, Baptista P, Correia D, et al. "Effects of Conservation Treatment and Cooking on the Chemi-cal Composition and Antioxidant Activity of Portuguese Wild Edible Mushrooms." *Journal of Agriculture and Food Chemistry.* **2007:***55* (12),

pgs 4781–4788. Link LB, Potter JD. "Raw versus cooked vegetables and cancer risk." *Cancer Epidemiology, Biomarkers & Prevention.* 2004: 13(9):1422-35.

15 Jackson LS, Al-Taher F. "Effects of consumer food preparation on acrylamide formation." *Advances in Experimental Medicine and Biology.* 2005:561:447-65. Halton TL, Willett WC, Liu S, et al. "Potato and French fry consumption and risk of type 2 diabetes in women." *American Journal of Clinical Nutrition.* 2006 Feb;83(2):284-90.

16 Lubec G, Wolf C, Bartosh B. "Amino acid isomerisation and microwave exposure." *Lancet.* 2(8676):1392-93, 1989 87.

17 Acrylamide Facts. http://www.acrylamidefacts.org/faqs.aspx. Accessed 10/14/10.

18 Grinder-Pederson L, Rasmussen SE, Bugel S, et al. "Effect of diets based on foods from conventional versus organic production on intake and excretion of flavonoids and markers of antioxidative defense in humans." *Journal of Agriculture and Food Chemistry.* 2003:51(19): 5671-5676.

19 Cheney, Garnett M.D. "Rapid Healing of Peptic Ulcers in patients Receiving Fresh Cabbage Juice." *California Medicine.* Vol. 70, No. 1. Pgs 10-15. January 1949.

20 Walker, N.W. *Raw Vegetable Juices.* New York: Pyramid Books. 1972.

21 Craig WJ, PhD, MPH, RD, and Mangels AR, PhD, RD, LDN, FADA. "Position of the American Dietetic Association: Vegetarian Diets." *Journal of the American Dietetic Association.* 2009:109:1266-1282.

22 North American Vegetarian Society. *Vegetarian FAQ.* www.navs-online.org/faq/index.php. Accessed 6/09/10.

23 Tucker, K. L., M. T. Hannan, H. Chen, et al. "Potassium, magnesium and fruit and vegetable intakes are associated with greater bone mineral density in elderly men and women." *American Journal of Clinical Nutrition.* 68(4): 727-36. 1999. Hu JF, Zhao XH, Parpia B, et al. 1993. "Dietary intakes and urinary excretion of calcium and acids: a cross-sectional study of women in China." *American Journal of Clinical Nutrition.* 1993:58 (3): 398 – 406.

24 Fuhrman, J. *Eat to Live*. New York: Little, Brown and Company. 2003. Pgs 88-90.

25 Hegsted DM. "Calcium and osteoporosis." *Journal of Nutrition*. 1986. 116:2316-9.

Chapter Five

1 Organisation for Economic Co-operation and Development. "OECD Health at a Glance 2009: Key findings for the United States." Organization for Economic Co-operation and Development. http://tinyurl.com/oecd-healthstats. Website accessed 05/26/10.

2 Campbell TC, Campbell, TM. *The China Study*. Dallas, Texas: Benbella Books. 2006. Page 109-110.

3 Mozafar A. "Enrichment of some B-vitamins in plants with application of organic fertilizers." *Plant and Soil*. 1994: 167: 305-311.

4 Petersen KF, et al. "Impaired Mitochyondrial Activity in the Insulin-Resistant Offspring of Patients with Type 2 Diabetes." *New England Journal of Medicine*. 2004: 350: 664-71. Greco AV, et al. "Insulin Resistance in Morbid Obesity: Reversal with Intramyocellular Fat Depletion." *Diabetes*. 2002: 52: 144-51 Goff LM, et al. "Veganism and Its Relationship with Insulin Resistance and Intramyocellular Lipid." *European Journal of Clinical Nutrition*. 2005: 59: 291-8. Barnard, Neal. *Dr. Neal Barnard's Program for Reversing Diabetes*. New York: Rodale. 2007.

5 Esselstyn, Caldwell B. Jr., M.D. *Prevent and Reverse Heart Disease*. New York: Penguin Group (USA) Inc. 2007.

6 Barnard, Neal M.D. *Breaking the Food Seduction*. New York: St. Martin's Press. 2003.

Chapter Six

1 Brimner, J. Douglas. *Before You Take That Pill*. New York: The Penguin Group (USA) Inc. 2008.

2 Abramson, John M.D. *Overdosed American: The Broken Promise of American Medicine*. New York: HarperCollins Publishers, Inc. 2004.

3 Robinson, Malcolm K. M.D. "Surgical Treatment of Obesity—Weighing the Facts." *The New England Journal of Medicine.* 2009; 361: 520-521. July 30, 2009. www.nejm.org/doi/pdf/10.1056/NEJMe0904837. Accessed 08/25/10.

4 American Society for Gastrointestinal Endoscopy. "Press Release: Endoscopy Identified as Safe and Effective Method in Treating Common Complication of Gastric Bypass Surgery." August 16, 2007. www.asge. org/PressroomIndex.aspx?id=3632. Accessed 08/25/10.

5 Maynard C, Goss JR, Malenka DJ, et al. "Adjusting for Patient Differences in Predicting Hospital Mortality for Percutaneous Coronary Intervention in the Clinical Outcomes Assessment Program." *American Heart Journal.* www.medscape.com/viewarticle/452792. Accessed 08/25/10.

Chapter Seven
1 Fuhrman, Joel, M.D. *Eat For Health, Book One.* Flemington: Joel Fuhrman, MD. 2008. Pgs 51-55.

Chapter Nine
1 American Heart Association. "Blood Pressure Levels." http://www. americanheart.org/presenter.jhtml?identifier=4450. Accessed 9/17/10.

2 American Heart Association. "Resting Heart Rate." http://www.americanheart.org/presenter.jhtml?identifier=4701. Accessed 9/17/10.

3 Cleveland Clinic. "Inflammation: What You Need to Know." http://my.clevelandclinic.org/symptoms/inflammation/hic_inflammation_what_you_need_to_know.aspx. Accessed 9/17/10.

4 Life Extension. "Inflammation: Chronic." http://www.lef.org/protocols/prtcls-txt/t-prtcl-146.html. Accessed 9/17/10.

5 Ridker PM, Cushman M, Stampfer M.J, et al. "Inflammation, aspirin, and the risk of cardiovascular disease in apparently healthy men." *The New England Journal of Medicine.* 1997. Jul31;337(5):356.

6 Ridker PM, Danielson E., Fonesca F AH, et al. "Rosuvastatin to Prevent Vascular Events in Men and Women with Elevated C-Reactive Protein." *The New England Journal of Medicine.* 2008:359 (21):2195-2207.

7 American Heart Association. "Good vs. Bad Cholesterol." http:// www.heart.org/EARTORG/Conditions/Cholesterol/AboutCholesterol/ Good-vs-Bad-Cholesterol_UCM_305561_Article.jsp. Accessed 9/17/10.

8 American Heart Association. "What Your Cholesterol Levels Mean." http://www.heart.org/HEARTORG/Conditions/Cholesterol/About Cholesterol/What-Your-Cholesterol-Levels-Mean_UCM_305562_ Article.jsp. Accessed 09/20/10.

9 American Diabetes Association. "American Diabetes Association's New Clinical Practice Recommendations Promote AIC as Diagnostic Test for Diabetes." December 29, 2009. www.diabetes.org/for-media/2009/cpr-2010-a1cdiagnostic-tool.html. Accessed 9/16/10.

10 RnCeus.com. "Blood Urea Nitrogen (BUN)." http://rnceus.com/renal/ renalbun.html. Accessed 9/16/10.

11 RnCeus.com. "Serum Creatinine." http://rnceus.com/renal/renalcreat. html. Accessed 9/16/10.

Chapter Ten

1 Racette SB, Schoeller DA, Kushner RF, et al. "Exercise enhances dietary compliance during moderate energy restriction in obese women." *American Journal of Clinical Nutrition*. 1995: 62:345-9.

Index

CPSIA information can be obtained at www.ICGtesting.com
Printed in the USA
BVOW05s1851040314

346648BV00012B/384/P